CARER SUPPORT IN THE COMMUNITY

EVALUATION OF THE DEPARTMENT OF HEALTH INITIATIVE: 'DEMONSTRATION DISTRICTS FOR INFORMAL CARERS' 1986-1989

COMPILED BY DIONE HILLS,
TAVISTOCK INSTITUTE OF
HUMAN RELATIONS

DEPARTMENT OF HEALTH

SOCIAL SERVICES INSPECTORATE

First published 1991
ISBN 0 11 321365 4

The work was commissioned by the Department of Health but the authors are responsible for statements made and the views and opinions expressed, which are not necessarily those of the Department of Health or HMSO.

Foreword by the Rt Hon Lady Seear

The story of "care in the community" over the last 30 years has recurrently been one of expectations raised and then dashed. It began in the late 1950s, when the 1959 Mental Health Act promoted the winding down of the big long-stay hospitals for mentally ill handicapped people. The argument was strong: institutionalization itself worsened the conditions for which patients had originally been admitted; the best route to normalisation and possibly rehabilitation was through sheltered accommodation and the back-up of professional resources in the community. Half-way houses began to be established. For somewhat similar reasons, long-stay geriatric wards were seen to be inappropriate places for younger people suffering from physical disabilities or chronic illnesses but mentally alert. Many of these moved out into voluntary homes and local authority establishments. Apart from the sound reasons for decanting long-stay patients, there was also undoubtedly a hope that the community alternative would be cheaper. Though clearly unfounded, this hope still lingers, and "community care", so called, has been chronically under-resourced. Particularly in the case of mental illness, the results are all to visible on the streets today.

Meanwhile, the demand for long-stay beds in hospitals and residential homes actually increased. This was partly due to a shift in social values: instead of "the family should look after its own", there was a growing demand that the Welfare State should provide. This was exacerbated by demographic and social changes: the rising proportion of older people; more mobility; more women in employment; more broken families. The number of potential carers of dependent family members was declining. In the mid-1970s, policy studies were beginning to foresee an escalating demand for statutory care.

In this context, "informal carers" gradually became recognized as a significant resource; and they themselves were making their voices heard. Many carers of all ages wanted" to look after their own", but they needed help to do so.

The 1985 General Household survey revealed the extent of the problem.

Fifteen per cent of women and twelve per cent of men carried the main responsibility for domestic care of a sick, handicapped or elderly person, usually a close relative. In the general population, this would mean six million people. Three per cent (about 2.2 million) were devoting a minimum of 20 hours a week to caring. And these figures do not include carers under 16, of whom there are known to be many. Not surprisingly, the Griffiths Report in 1988 urged that separate recognition should be given to carers' needs and this was reinforced by the White Paper.

The question, so far unanswered, has been: What kinds of support are most helpful and appropriate for what kinds of carers? It is here that this new report from the Tavistock Institute of Human Relations makes an important contribution. Through careful evaluation of some 50 schemes run by voluntary organizations, coupled with surveys and individual interviews with carers, it offers a much clearer picture of carers' needs and the packages of services that may help them. It also gives us a salutary reminder that reliability and humanity in service provision can be just as important as the content of the support that is given.

There is much here that will be valuable for planners and managers in the social services and also in the health service and the voluntary sector. Current financial constraints make it vital that the funds that are available should be spent wisely and well. There is some good news in the report: quite modest supports can make a big difference to a carers' morale and health. However, it also tells us that, whilst there are good social grounds for helping carers to sustain heavily dependent family members at home, it requires substantial resources. So the myth of community care as the cheap option is once again exploded.

Preface and Acknowledgements

This publication provides a summary of the findings from a programme funded by the Department of Health, called 'Demonstration Districts for Informal Carers'. In each of three local authority areas, voluntary consortia were established to distribute grants to voluntary organisations that undertook to set up or run services for carers.

The publication is designed particularly for managers and policy makers in social services departments and health services, as well as those in the voluntary sector, who are considering the role of the voluntary sector in care in the community, and particularly in the support of carers looking after people with disabilities at home. It was compiled by one of the researchers funded to evaluate the programme, in conjunction with Sharon Haffenden, a senior development officer employed by one of the consortia, and Dr. Eric Miller, research consultant at the Tavistock Institute of Human Relations. A companion volume has also been produced by Sharon Haffenden, which draws on the experience gained in the three districts to provide a practical guide for workers and managers wishing to develop services.

A central feature of this programme was the active participation in the evaluation of all those involved: consortia members, workers employed by the consortia, management committees and workers in the voluntary organisations funded to provide services to carers, and members of the Department of Health Social Services Inspectorate. In being involved in this, each has contributed in an important way to the production of this publication. Particular mention should be made of the contribution of the three chairs of the consortia: Fred Smith, Andy Hutchings and Joan Cooper, and of the other employees of the consortia: Roger Page, Paul Endersby, Jane Brotchie, David Sutcliffe, Sandy Lazarus, Wendy Wallace and Lucette Tucker.

Three of the evaluation reports produced locally have been included in their entirety as appendices to the summary of the main findings in this publication; other material from the programme can be found in the publications listed below and in journal articles referred to in the text.

Other documents referred to in this publication are available as follows:

Getting it Right for Carers: Sharon Haffenden. HMSO 1991

Demonstration Districts Final Research Report (and associated working papers): Tavistock Institute of Human Relations. 120 Belsize Lane, London NW3 5BA

East Sussex Evaluation Report: Carers' Council, 143 High St, Lewes, East Sussex. BN7 1XT

Sandwell Child Carer Report: Sandwell Carers Centre, 2 Bearwood Rd, Smethwick, W. Midlands.

CONTENTS

INTRODUCTION

This report provides a brief account of an experiment set up by the Department of Health to look at new ways in which the voluntary sector could provide support for carers. The findings of this experiment are timely, as social services and the voluntary sector face the task of supporting a growing population of people with physical and mental disabilities within the community.

The key role of carers in provision of care in the community has gradually come to be recognised by professionals and policy makers over the last 5 years. The Disabled Persons Act (1986) has sections that require social services departments to take into account the ability of carers to provide care when assessing the needs of people with disabilities. The new community care approach asks local authorities to design the packages of services tailored to meet the assessed needs of both individuals (with disabilities) and their carers.

However, in seeking to provide services for carers, many local authorities will face a dearth of suitable services. Although the voluntary sector has taken a key role in developing support and information services, respite and relief care for carers, provision in most places is still patchy. The new community care legislation places a responsibility on social services departments to help the non-statutory agencies to develop new services, so the question of how to encourage the growth of suitable new services in the voluntary sector will become an issue of increasing importance.

The programme described in this report addresses this issue. Part of the Department of Health's 'Helping the Community to Care' Initiative, the 'Demonstration Districts for Informal Carers' programme established consortia in three local authority areas. These in turn funded voluntary organisations to provide a range of support services for carers provided by voluntary organisations. The availability of grant aid enabled voluntary agencies to experiment with new forms of support.

Over the three years of the programme, each of the consortia (in East

Sussex, Sandwell and Stockport) had a budget of £200,000 a year to spend on grants to local voluntary agencies, and on developmental activities to promote awareness of carers or to help in the establishment of new agencies and new services. As well as establishing new activities, they were also asked to monitor these and help to share the lessons learned with others. Guidelines sent out by the Department of Health described the task as follows:

> i. to enhance developments and promote new initiatives in the voluntary sector in supporting informal carers in specific local authority areas, in order to demonstrate the value of these,
>
> ii. to provide reports for use in other areas to promote support for informal carers, and engage with other developments on a wider front, and
>
> iii. to monitor and identify outcomes and indicators for the future in terms of support for carers.

The task of monitoring was shared with the Tavistock Institute of Human Relations, which was funded to evaluate the programme. In this the Institute worked alongside the consortia and the Department of Health, supporting self evaluation at all levels, and helping in the production of reports and dissemination of material. This led to a whole range of 'outputs' from the programme apart from a final research report: local evaluation reports, discussion papers, a video, two national conferences and several articles in newspapers and journals.

For ease of access, this material has been brought together in two publications. This one provides a brief summary of the whole programme, outlining the main findings, giving references to other reports and articles produced during the three years. It focuses particularly on the developmental aspects of the programme: the effectiveness of different strategies in grant distribution, and the resources required for the development of new services. It also contains three reports produced by the consortia which give details of the services established in their area, information about the characteristics of carers using these and carers' evaluation of the services.

A second publication; 'Getting it Right for Carers', provides practical guidance, based on the experience gained in this programme, for those in statutory and voluntary organisations wishing to set up new services for carers, and a wealth of information to assist with each stage in the development of new services. It also provides a range of different models of services, together with comments on the relative advantages and disadvantages of each, and indications of the kind of resources that they will require. It is also available from H.M.S.O.

SOME KEY POINTS EMERGING FROM THE EVALUATION

◆ Stimulating the voluntary sector

● Each of the three consortia, which brought together representatives of key voluntary and statutory agencies, successfully distributed a budget of £200,000 a year in grants to local voluntary agencies and provided an important stimulus to the development of new services and of promotional and campaigning activities on behalf of carers.

● 43 new services for carers were developed by a variety of different agencies, from large professional voluntary organisations to small carer self help groups. 35 of these, with the backing of the consortia, were able to find local sources of funding, mostly from local statutory sources, after the Department of Health initiative funding came to an end.

◆ The role of a local consortium

● Members of the consortia reported an increased understanding of carer issues within their organisations, and an increase in collaboration and joint working between agencies involved in the provision of support to carers. Some felt that co-operation and mutual understanding between voluntary and statutory sectors had also improved. However, there was little evidence that local voluntary agencies that did not receive grants (even if represented on the consortium) were stimulated to develop new services for carers.

◆ The grant giving strategy

● Although a mainly reactive grant giving strategy was tried in two districts, it was soon apparent that demand was exceeding supply, and more specific criteria for grant allocation and priorities were needed. A reactive strategy would probably not have met the full range of carers' needs: in all districts there were needs that local voluntary agencies did not immediately come forward with services to meet: including information and advice needs, night sitting services, services for carers of people with mental health problems and the needs of ethnic minority carers.

- A more focused strategy, based on an assessment of the needs of carers in the area and the gaps in existing services, enabled consortia staff to take a more proactive role in encouraging specific voluntary organisations to set up services to meet the needs identified. In some cases, consortia staff encouraged new branches of national voluntary organisations to become established in the areas, and helped establish a small number of new organisations to provide services that existing organisations were less interested in developing.

- Larger and well established voluntary organisations were in the best position to respond quickly to the availability of grant aid: smaller, more informal agencies often needed help in preparing applications. In areas where the voluntary sector is small and fragmented (eg in rural areas), few services would have developed without a considerable input of developmental time by consortia staff.

◆ The role of consortia staff

- In each district consortia appointed staff who undertook developmental activities, increasing awareness of carers and their needs amongst professionals and public, supporting the grant aided services that were established, and developing new networks or activities where gaps had been identified.

- Monitoring and evaluation were important aspects of the work of the consortia, undertaken primarily by consortia staff, with guidance from the Tavistock Institute researchers. This enabled consortia to pick up problems in schemes at an early stage, and help to remedy these. Some agencies ran into internal difficulties when establishing their services, particularly where they lacked experience in recruiting and managing paid staff. Others had difficulty in getting the cooperation of professionals and in contacting carers in need of services.

- Effective monitoring systems developed by the funded schemes and the awareness raising work undertaken by consortia staff, played an important role in enabling services to obtain further funding.

◆ The services set up

● Most services primarily addressed the needs of the carers themselves although a few focused on the person cared for on the assumption that the carer would also benefit. The benefit felt by carers was more limited in the latter cases.

● Organisations in which carers were involved tended to favour home based relief care services (in which care attendants looked after their dependant at home), information, advice and support services.

● The majority of grant-aided services employed paid staff, with around half being run entirely by paid staff. Around a third used a combination of staff and volunteers.

● Many of the services grant aided had been tried elsewhere, but were not yet available for carers in these areas. Some existing services sought resources to expand to a wider range of carers. However, a number of innovative services were also developed, including carer support workers, specialist 'carer resource and information centres', and services in which the primary support was provided by volunteers, 'good neighbours', and other carers.

● Specially designed carer resource centres were seen as one solution to carers' information and advice needs, and each district developed a different model. All three had considerable success in contacting carers, particularly those in an early stage of caring, but there were difficulties in finding funding for these centres from local sources.

◆ Carers' response to services

● Services supported by grants reached around 10% of carers in the three districts. They tended to reach those who were in great need of support, because of age, stress, ill health, or level of dependency of the person they were looking after.

● Carers' need for services could not be judged just by the dependency of the person they were looking after. In many cases, it was the age and frailty of the carers themselves that was a key issue.

● Carers on the whole were very well satisfied with the services that were provided by the voluntary sector, and saw these as being helpful in a variety of ways (see section 3). They saw the workers as being particularly helpful and understanding of their situation. This contrasted with criticism of other services (often statutory services) particularly those orientated towards the needs of their dependants.

◆ Use of volunteers

- Volunteers were able to provide a valuable service to carers, particularly when they were familiar with the problems that the carers were experiencing (eg had also had relatives or friends suffering from cancer or schizophrenia). However, in most cases, services using volunteers tended to cater for carers whose dependants were less heavily handicapped than those employing paid care staff.

- Schemes using volunteers were not much cheaper to run than fully staffed services. The input from coordinators was higher, per carer, where volunteers were the main service providers.

◆ Cost of services

- The overall cost of many of the services was quite low (the majority cost between £10,000 and £25,000 a year, 1987 prices), but the true cost was sometimes masked by the fact that they were receiving support in kind from other agencies (eg free accommodation). However, at the end of the three years, in most cases it proved impossible to cover these costs from charitable fund raising, donations or from trust funds. Despite efforts in these directions, most services had to rely on funding from either health authorities, social service departments or joint finance in order to keep their services to carers running.

1 NEEDS OF CARERS

Characteristics of carers:

Policy on community care is based on the assumption that people with long term disabilities or illness would prefer to live for as long as possible in their own home, with appropriate support. In many cases, the main source of support comes from family members, but the capacity of family members to provide care can vary. For many carers, support is provided only at a cost to themselves, ie. cost of lost employment opportunities, lost financial security, or physical and mental ill health. The extent to which they are able to continue to provide care can sometimes depend on the level of services provided to the disabled person or to themselves.

The difficulty that many carers have in coping was shown clearly in the surveys of carers receiving voluntary services carried out in East Sussex and Sandwell (1) (2):

- 70% of the carers were women. In East Sussex half were over 65, and nearly a quarter were over 75 years old. Two thirds of the people they were looking after were over 65.

- most (89%) said that they spent 50 hours or more caring each week: three quarters were unable to leave their dependants without someone looking after them, and two thirds said that it would be difficult to find anyone else to stand in for them.

- three quarters had health problems of their own: other problems included difficulty in lifting, bathing and toileting their dependants, isolation, inability to get out to do shopping or see other family members, lack of information about services, lack of sleep, constant worry and stress, and doubts about being able to carry on.

- most had been caring for five years or more; a quarter had been caring for over 10 years.

Carers' needs for services:

For many carers, the most obvious need is for some kind of practical help with the physical tasks of caring and for regular breaks in order to do the things that the demands of caring make difficult: to take a rest, to attend to their own health or interests, to keep in touch with friends and other family members, or just undertake basic household tasks such as shopping.

In addition to practical help, many carers also have needs for emotional support, advice and information. 28 carers using voluntary services were interviewed in depth: few of these were able to undertake paid work, and many were unaware of all the benefits to which they were entitled. Emotional strain came from the shock of discovery of the illness or disability of their dependant, coping with the changed personality and relationship (particularly with elderly dementing relatives), constant guilt, frustration at the restriction of their lives, and anger, at their dependant relative or other family members or services that were giving them no support.

While most wished to carry on caring as long as they were able, lack of suitable alternatives to family care meant that some continued caring in spite of their own deteriorating physical and mental health, with a constant anxiety about 'what would happen if anything happened to me'. (3)

A high proportion of carers using the voluntary services set up in the three demonstration districts were in older age groups, and looking after very dependent people. The proportion unable to leave their dependants was higher than that in the General Household survey of carers undertaken by OPCS, (4), and they were more often looking after people with mental disabilities as well as physical ones. Many of the carers using the voluntary schemes were already receiving some support from statutory services, (1) (2), financial assistance, help from their GPs, from nurses, respite care, home helps or meals on wheels.

Although many described these services as helpful, a number also expressed frustration with the limitations of these. The services were usually directed at the needs of the person that they were looking after, and the carers' needs for help were often ignored. Indeed, sometimes the way that services were provided added to the carers' stress rather than relieving it, particularly where they felt that they had to fight to get help. Other irritants were:

- the lack of information about likely prognosis and appropriate care of their dependants or about other services in the locality that might have made the caring task easier,

- unreliability of the service (eg., late arrival of transport services to take their dependant to daycentre meant that carers couldn't plan their own activities around these),

- services provided too infrequently (eg., a weekly incontinence service allowed a build up of soiled bedclothes in the home),

- services that did not meet the needs of the dependant (eg., meals on wheels that didn't take into account differing cultural tastes), and

- services that led to the distress of their dependant or a deterioration in their condition, through poor levels of care, disruption of regular routines and resulting disorientation (eg. respite care) (3).

Sensitivity of those providing services to the carers' situation can be crucial to a successful intervention. Because many carers feel guilty at asking for help at all, the reliability of care and the acceptability of the services to their dependant were often key factors in their decisions about whether to use a service or not. (3)

This means that services must be adaptable to the needs of both carers and those they were looking after. One service in itself is rarely sufficient, and a package of support is frequently needed in order to reduce the stress in any given situation. Carers' needs can be highly specific, and can change as the overall situation develops: there may be a need for both long and short term breaks, help at particularly stressful times such as during the night (lack of sleep is a major cause of stress) as well as practical help and emotional support at times when it is needed. Because caring is a 24 hour, 7 day a week task, crises can often occur outside office hours.

Although useful in some cases, standardised and written information may be insufficient; carers frequently need help in sorting out what are their central needs, and what kind of service would make their particular situation more manageable. Information and advice at the onset of disability or illness of their dependant were particularly important, but some carers also need help after their dependant dies, since for many years they may have built their lives around the needs of others.

Child carers:

A survey of secondary schools in Sandwell showed that teachers knew of at least 95 children of secondary school age in the borough (total population of secondary school age is 19,000) who had primary responsibility for a sick or handicapped family member. A further 74 children were thought to be carers. Around half of the children were under 14. About a third were felt to be underattaining educationally. Other problems included isolation from friends, stress, worry and poor concentration, lateness and poor attendance and lack of parental support. Intervention in these situations is a particularly sensitive issue, since there is a real danger of breaking up the family. Teachers lacked information about how they could help these children (5), but in this they did not differ greatly from many professionals who come into contact with carers, who may themselves not be aware of services (particularly when these are provided by a variety of agencies) in their area.

Carers from ethnic minority groups:

Few carers from ethnic minority groups were to use the services set up in the three Demonstration Districts, apart from one, specialist service for Asian families. There were indications that carers from minority groups found it difficult to use services in which care attendants, volunteers, host families and other carers came from a different cultural group. Apart from language difficulties, caring involves intimate contact in which differing cultural expectations can be very important. This suggests that either specialist services should be set up, or that greater efforts are made to employ workers from the same cultural group.

No ethnic minority groups received grants to set up carer services in the Demonstration Districts: where there were active ethnic organisations, the orientation was towards general issues of cultural representation rather than community care, and attaching carer services to these would have required a major change in emphasis. Because of the speed with which most of the grants were distributed; there was little time to do the intensive development work that might have been required to help develop new services in this area.

There were major difficulties in contacting carers from minority groups: a lack of understanding of English made it hard for these carers to get information about services that they might have used. Often they were not in touch with even basic services: the scheme for Asian parents of handicapped children found many families with considerable difficulties which were unknown to the social service department. Sometimes there were cultural factors that made it difficult for carers in these groups to acknowledge handicaps in the family or to accept intervention from outside the immediate family.

Additional information from:

1. Appendix B
2. Appendix C
3. Demonstration Districts: final research report: Dione Hills with Eric Miller. Tavistock Institute of Human Relations 1990.
4. Informal Carers: Hazel Green (General Household Survey 1985) OPCS. 1988.
5. Child Carer Report: Sandwell Caring for Carers Project in conjunction with Sandwell MBC Education Department. Available from Sandwell Caring for Carers.

2 LOCAL CARER CONSORTIA: STRUCTURES AND STRATEGIES

When the Demonstration District Programme was first set up, it was thought that a local development agency, such as a local Council of Voluntary Service, would administer the grant distribution locally. However it was clear that there were a number of major local organisations that had an interest in, and some knowledge of services for, carers in each district, so in each case, a new body was established to undertake the work. Membership of the consortia set up included representatives of national voluntary organisations as well as local agencies, representatives of local statutory social services and health services, and a member of the Regional Social Services Inspectorate in an advisory role. A small number of carers were also invited to be part of each consortia.

The conditions attached to the Department of Health funding were open enough to allow for considerable local variation both in the structure of the consortia and the kind of policy adopted towards allocation of grants. The main conditions were that the grants awarded had to benefit carers and that they could go only to properly constituted voluntary organisations. While the whole programme was intended to be innovative, the consortia were encouraged to fund a mixture of innovative and tried and tested approaches to carer support. The consortia were allowed to use some of their funds to employ staff to assist them in their work, and two of them were to use this as an opportunity to employ staff to undertake major developmental roles.

East Sussex

East Sussex is a large county with a mixture of urban and rural areas. Although in some areas the voluntary sector was well developed and able to respond to the invitation to apply for grants, in other, rural, areas, there were few local organisations of any size. Partly for this reason, the consortium decided to set aside a large part of their funds (37%) for developmental activities. Two subcommittees were set up, one to oversee the development activities and one to administer the rest of the funds in grants. Both committees had decision-making powers over their own budget, only decisions over major grants being referred to the whole consortium. Meetings of the whole consortium could happen relatively infrequently (quarterly), which reflected the large size of the county and distances that some members had to travel. Three members were representatives of national organisations, invited onto the consortium to provide experience of carer issues. There was high level representation from the social services department.

The development funds were used to employ three workers: one full-time worker to cover the whole county, one part-time worker to cover a rural area, and a part-time training officer. In addition, the consortium had a coordinator seconded by the Social Services Department and a full time administrative post.

The goals of the development staff, after an initial period of research into carers need in the county, were:

- to create change in attitude towards carers,
- to create opportunities for people working with carers to come together,
- to enable the development of projects to co-ordinate services for carers, and
- to provide training and information on aspects of caring and carers' needs.

The strategy adopted by the grants committee was initially a responsive one: each application considered on its own merit. However, it was soon clear that the criteria by which decisions were being made needed to be clarified, in order to help organisations planning an application. The criteria adopted were that:

- the money should be spread across the county ensuring that rural areas received their share,
- schemes should give direct services to carers (rather than indirect, via services to their dependants), and
- schemes should be innovative – that is, a new way of delivering an established service, a new recipient group or a new combination of services.

Monitoring and evaluation fell under the responsibility of the grant sub-committee and was undertaken by the two full time workers. (1)

Stockport:

In Stockport the voluntary sector was large and well developed, with a long history of collaboration with the local statutory services. There were a number of active carer groups in the borough. The consortium was made up of: representatives of large local voluntary organisations, several of which were already involved in providing some support to carers, the assistant director from the Social Services Department, and representatives from health services. The Treasurer's Department was to provide help to both the consortium and some of the grant aided organisations with accounting and financial administration.

The consortium brought together its collective experience early in the programme in a day workshop. Out of this came a strategy that emphasised the development of services to meet a range of carers' needs, and to target those carers most in need of support. Previous research had shown that it was often carers who were looking after people with the heaviest handicaps that received the least support. The identified needs of the carers were for:

- information and advice about caring,
- recognition from professional carers,
- practical help,
- regular respite,
- emotional support and psychological insight.

The two (part-time) workers appointed by the consortium undertook the developmental task of identifying local organisations interested in providing services to meet these needs and working with these organisations to help them develop new services. They also undertook evaluation, and, with the consortium, addressed the problem of professional recognition and support of carers through a programme of education and training, information fairs, and a promotional video. Later they helped schemes to secure continuing funding.

An important feature of the Stockport consortium was involvement of carer members, particularly the efforts taken to ensure their full participation in the two subcommittees. These were set up to deal with grant applications, and with research and monitoring: membership was rotated every three meetings to ensure that every one had a chance to participate actively. However, the subcommittees were advisory: decisions were taken at the full committee meetings every two months. The research and monitoring subcommittee played a key role in the evaluation of services, with the workers being directly involved in helping the schemes to evaluate their own activities.

Sandwell:

Like some parts of East Sussex, much of the voluntary sector in Sandwell was small and localised, with little experience at running major services. Few organisations had previous experience of running services for carers and, partly for this reason, it was decided to invite several representatives of national organisations onto the consortium. The consortium had also close political links with the council, with the chair of the Social Services Committee undertaking chairmanship of the consortium. It also sought to work in close collaboration with officers from local statutory services.

The consortium was keen to see its resources distributed directly to voluntary organisations that could provide practical services to carers, and developmental work took a relatively low priority. However, several of the consortium members were in key developmental roles in their organisations (as regional developmental workers for national agencies, or development workers in local agencies) and these had an important role in the establishment of new carer services within their agencies.

On the whole, the grant aiding strategy adopted was a responsive one, putting the onus on the applicants for grants to make the case for the services that they wanted to develop. The main developmental work of the staff member (director) appointed in the early stages was work with some of the smaller organisations, to help them draw up constitutions and prepare their applications to the consortium, and work with ethnic minority organisations. This strategy led to the establishment of several new agencies in the borough and a major change in direction for some of the existing agencies. They also funded a major project providing support to Asian families with handicapped children. Together with the Education Department they also undertook a survey of the number and needs of school children who were carers.

Although eschewing a more general developmental role, the consortium held several public meetings to bring carers to the attention of service agencies in the borough, and worked through their links with the Social Services Department to secure future funding for the schemes. As the consortium wanted to retain full decision-making powers, it did not set up a subcommittee, although an executive committee handled some of the day by day managerial functions. One full-time officer was appointed, with secretarial support, to service the consortium. Evaluation reports were compiled by the director in collaboration with schemes and reviewed by the consortium as a whole.

Effectiveness of Structure:

Although the three consortia had very different structures to manage and distribute their funds, a survey undertaken part way through the last year showed that most consortia members were reasonably satisfied, which suggests that each found the right model to fit its particular political and geographical circumstances (2). It also showed that similar difficulties emerged, whatever the model chosen. Subcommittees had clearly provided a useful forum for more detailed discussions about carers' needs, and helped members to feel more directly involved in the day to day work, but they also led some members to feel excluded from 'real' decision making. In all three districts some members felt that their skills and knowledge had not been fully utilised.

Another concern expressed in all three districts was that carers did not feel fully involved in consortia activities. Although steps were taken to recruit carers as members, many felt that the size and style of meetings made it difficult for these to contribute. Members also found consortium business made heavy demands on their time, which was particularly difficult if they were employees of other agencies. Many gave both personal and work time to consortia business, which, they estimated, averaged to be around one and a half days a month.

Effectiveness of Strategy:

Although most members were satisfied with the outcome of their consortia in terms of the services set up, some felt that there had been undue pressure in the early stages to allocate grants, and insufficient time to plan properly and establish priorities in their grant allocation. Because of the lack of alternative sources of funding locally for services for carers, schemes set up during the first year remained largely dependent on consortium funds throughout the three years, which meant that the decisions made in the first year determined the pattern of allocation for the three years. Setting aside funds for development activities gave East Sussex greater scope for funding new and innovative services established with the help of the development workers. A rigorous approach to monitoring enabled the Stockport consortium to redistribute some of its funding in the second and third years, and to fund new services set up with the help of the development worker. Sandwell kept a small part of its funding back to distribute for small grants later in the programme.

Strategically, all three consortia ran into some difficulty around the distribution of funding within the financial year since it was unclear at first whether funds granted in one year could be carried over into the next. Several projects took longer to establish than expected, but expectations were sometimes unrealistic: the average set up time, of around 3 months, was very reasonable.

In retrospect several people felt that a more flexible funding arrangement, with less money available in the first year, would have been more manageable. Several members also felt that more staff time could have been allocated in all three districts, although in the early days, many were keen to see as little as possible spent on administration. As time went on, it was apparent that many of the services, particularly if run by small or newly established organisations, needed help in resolving a number of practical and managerial problems. Monitoring the grants allocated and evaluating services was also time consuming, but an important activity, both as a means of ensuring that grants were being spent effectively and as an opportunity to pick up any problems arising. It also provided an important point at which representatives from other agencies were kept informed about the developing services, facilitating inter agency cooperation.

The importance of campaigning and promotional work also became more apparent as time passed, and it became clear that raising funds to continue carer services after the end of the Department of Health funding, was going to be far from easy.

Additional information from:

1. East Sussex Evaluation Report
2. Final Research report from the Tavistock Institute

3 SERVICES FOR CARERS

Voluntary organisations in the three demonstration districts came up with a wide variety of projects designed to provide support to carers. Some of these were services that had already been shown to be effective elsewhere, and some were innovative. For the most part grants were requested for ongoing services, although a few were requested for one-off activities such as a carer consultative meeting, or production of an information pack.

The kind of help provided to carers was very varied, but fell into four broad categories:

- **Alternative care for the dependant in the home**, so that the carer could take a break. These were mainly sitting services and respite care services; care was provided either by paid care attendants or volunteers. These services also provided some carers with help with the physically difficult tasks such as dressing and bathing of the dependant, or help at difficult times, such as getting a handicapped child dressed while their mother gets siblings ready for school.
- **Alternative care for the dependant away from home**, so that the carer could take a break. These included day centres, clubs (some for carer and dependant to attend together), schemes in which a 'host family' looked after the dependant for several days at a time, and schemes that provided, usually volunteer, companions who would take the dependant out.
- **Information and advice for the carers** about services, benefits and how to handle the caring situation. These included three 'carer resource centres', help lines, a CAB home visitor, information packs, and staff (carer support workers attached to other facilities with responsibility to advise and support carers).
- **Support and advocacy for carers**: sometimes this involves an opportunity for carers to talk to others about their situation, (emotional support) or just to meet with others socially (reducing isolation). These were provided by carer support groups, counselling services, carer support workers, and carer consultation workshops. A more active support role included activities closely related to case management, in which carer workers undertook t[illegible] help carers obtain and organise a range of services for themselves and th[illegible] dependants.

Although most schemes specialised in providing one of the above categories of help, some provided more than one kind. Some relief care schemes and information services also ran, or were run by, a carer group, or provided a coffee morning when carers could meet one another. Workers running practical services, such as sitting services, also provided advice and information to the carers referred to their service, and emotional support, such as bereavement care after the dependant died.

Although the consortia were anxious that services should be of direct benefit to carers themselves, some schemes provided this support via care for the dependant. This was particularly true of services that looked after the dependant away from home. These services had the advantage of providing dependants with new interests, reducing the pressure on the carer/dependant relationship. However, attendance at activities away from home relied on the good health of the dependant and their willingness to go out. Feedback from carers was harder to obtain on these services (they tended to see them as being provided for the dependants' benefit), and carers reported rather fewer benefits to themselves from using these.

None of the voluntary organisations in the three districts came up with schemes for residential respite services for carers (host family schemes were the closest that any came to this) nor night time sitting services (except occasionally in an emergency). Both are services that carers would have liked to have available.

Which organisations set up carer services?

Most schemes were set up by well established local voluntary agencies; about a third, like Age Concern, Crossroads, CVSs, were part of a national network; a further third were local groups that did not have this kind of back-up. A few grants went to national or regional agencies to establish new services in the area. Many grants went to agencies whose primary role had previously been support of people with disabilities, rather than their carers; setting up services for carers required some redirection of their focus and approach.

Organisations that were already undertaking work with carers were usually fairly new organisations (two or three years old). Some of these were carer groups or groups of 'friends' (often relatives and carers) of residential establishments. On the whole, carer groups asked for small grants to enable them to provide extensions to existing activities. Where they requested a major grant to set up a new service, they often required some new organisational structure to manage this. Young organisations and carer groups often had difficulties managing the changes required in developing services.

Some of the largest grants went to completely new organisations created specially to set up services funded by the consortia. Apart from new Crossroads Care Attendant schemes, which had support from their regional development workers, new organisations took longer than other schemes to get going, and received considerable help from the development workers employed by the consortia.

Cost of services:

Grants given varied between small amounts (£400–£1,000) given to enable carer groups to undertake some new activities, and large grants (up to £60,000) to establish major new services (for details of schemes and costs in each district, see appendices A–C). Most schemes employed paid workers; even if volunteers were providing the main services to carers, a paid worker usually provided the co-ordination. Salaries and supporting costs accounted for the main expenditure of most schemes; capital expenditure was usually confined to office equipment, although in two cases, buses were bought.

In most cases, grants from the consortia were the main source of funding for the service. However, many schemes received support in kind either from the voluntary agency that set them up, or from local health or social services departments, and this made an important difference to the overall cost. This was particularly true when the support provided was free use of premises, but other kinds of help included management of payroll, worker training, support and supervision and office services. Although in a few cases, management of the project was provided by a national or regional agency, for the most part it was provided by the volunteer management committee, often supplemented by a considerable input of voluntary time by the chair or a member of the committee with relevant experience.

Some of the services appear expensive because of the high costs of setting them up: this was particularly true when both the service and the organisation setting it up, were new, as in the case of the carer resource centres in the three districts. Running costs, particularly if calculated on a cost per carer basis, would probably have dropped in services such as the two host family schemes, but the short term nature of the programme made this hard to estimate. Day centres and host-family schemes were expensive but provided a longer period of respite for the carer than care attendant schemes. Care attendant schemes were more expensive when they catered for the elderly; this was partly because the turn-over of clients was higher, requiring more time to be given to assessment of new cases and support of bereaved carers.

Problems encountered:

Short term funding and the high profile of the project meant that schemes felt under pressure to get going quickly, and almost immediate pressure to find alternative sources of funding in order to continue after the DoH funds came to an end (1). Many of the organisations lacked experience in managing services or staff and several ran into internal management or organisational difficulties. In a few cases evaluation failed to show that carers were benefitting from services which were directed primarily at people with disabilities rather than their carers, or at the general public. Consortia staff intervened in some cases to help steer projects in the right direction, or to overcome their difficulties; but in eight cases projects were closed down after the initial grant had been used up (ie. a fifth of the projects that were intended to provide continuing services). In most of these cases only a small number of carers were using the service, but in several cases organisational problems had also been present.

The consortium in each district set up workshops at which staff and committee members from schemes could get together and discuss their services or a specific topic, such as fund raising. Most schemes have subsequently received offers of further funding from local sources (social services or health authority budgets, or joint finance); however, in all districts it required considerable time and energy by the consortia and their staff in order to ensure this funding in a climate where local budgets were already highly committed. The schemes that have had the greatest difficulty in all three districts have been the carer resource centres; these do not fit easily into the priorities of any local funding body and may be seen to be generating demands that statutory services are unable to meet. However, several research studies have shown that advice and information are a primary need for many carers.

A number of schemes had difficulties in recruiting and sometimes in keeping staff; this was partly because the short term nature of the programme created job insecurity, sometimes because levels of pay inadequately reflected the demands of work. Workers frequently found themselves undertaking hours and duties (eg fund raising) outside those laid down in job descriptions (2). Several schemes had difficulty recruiting volunteers. This was partly due to a general shortage of volunteers in the area. Many schemes also had difficulty in contacting carers and getting referrals from professional staff in statutory agencies. Especially in the early stages, considerable resources had to be devoted to publicity for services and ensuring that local statutory agencies were kept informed. Later on, many schemes became oversubscribed, and had to find ways of managing a waiting list, or rationing services in order to cope with the demand.

Users and their evaluation of services:

Around 4,500 carers have used the services funded in the three districts; some 10% of all carers completed questionnaires on the services they were receiving and a further 38 had in-depth interviews. A large proportion were caring for people with high levels of disability; there were also a high proportion of women, and of elderly carers. (3,4) One of the most marked features of the responses was the extent to which carers felt 'helped' on a number of different dimensions. Services were usually seen to be providing a variety of help outside their stated aims, and were appreciated for this; workers were described as 'very friendly', 'helpful', 'understanding', etc. Few carers made any criticism of the services they received, apart from wishing to receive more (relief care, etc.): this stands in contrast to the criticisms that carers sometimes make of statutory services. (See Section 2 and 5). The flexibility of the voluntary schemes, in being able to adapt themselves to the particular needs of individual carers, perhaps accounts for this high level of satisfaction, although an alternative view might be that carer expectations of voluntary services are lower than those they hold of statutory services. Carers frequently expressed their gratitude at receiving any help at all.

Innovative approaches to carer support:

Although the programme as a whole had been designed to encourage innovation in the voluntary sector, the overall paucity of services to carers meant that many of the grants were given to tried and tested models of carer support that were not yet available in the district. Examples of these were a Crossroad Care Attendant scheme and 'host family' scheme. Other grants were given to expand existing services so that more carers could benefit from them. For example, day centres were able to open at weekends, which are particularly stressful times for carers, and relief care services, which had previously had to limit the range of carers that they had been able to support because of limited funding, were able to cater for new categories of carer. Some grants went to establish more innovative and experimental schemes, including the three 'resource and information centres for carers' established in each district, appointments of specialist carer or family support workers attached to facilities for the handicapped or elderly, schemes for carers in rural areas, and innovative approaches to helping carers with the stress and emotional demands of caring. There were also experiments in the way services were provided: in volunteer services for carers, and in services that were run by the carers themselves.

Carer resource centres were well received by carers and professionals alike, professionals particularly appreciating 'one stop' to which they could refer for information about sources of help for carers. They reached a range of carers including those whose situation was not yet 'desperate' and who were unknown to other services providers. They were, however, expensive to set up and run, and all had difficulty in finding further funding from local sources in order to continue after the DoH funding ran out. They also all experienced problems with finding suitable premises, in finding suitable computer hard and software for their data bases, and in managing the varied expectations that different groups held about what they should do, and how they should run.

Counselling and emotional support for carers came in various guises. Attempts to provide a 'carer element' in general counselling services were not very successful; carers do not appear to be looking for counselling per se. However, counselling related to a particular illness was well accepted, as was the general support and help provided by carer support workers attached to other services, such as a day centre, or sitting service. Self-help projects such as the Carers Co-operative in East Sussex, in which carers of people with mental health problems helped others with similar problems, worked well, as did some of the carer groups and social activities such as 'coffee mornings' attached to other services.

Carer-run services. Some of these ran into serious difficulties because the management of a service was too much for a small inexperienced group already burdened with the demands of caring. However, with sufficient professional support and good paid workers, these were very successful. An attempt to run a 'creche' type of facility in which carers took turns at manning a Saturday club for dependants required considerable paid worker input, as well as considerable transport resources, which were difficult to sustain by the agency after DoH funding came to an end.

Volunteer run services. Services using volunteers were an attractive option because they are perceived to be an economic way of supporting carers, and to involve the community directly in the caring. Volunteers were successfully used in neighbourhood schemes, in sitting services, in providing companionship for handicapped young people, in family support where one member was a cancer sufferer and in carer resource centres. There were, however, limitations: services using volunteers tended to cater for carers with less heavily handicapped dependants (5). Some schemes had difficulty recruiting volunteers, particularly volunteers young and fit enough to cope with heavy lifting or pushing wheelchairs. Since, on the whole, one volunteer was attached to one carer, they could only cater for as many carers as there were volunteers. Demands on the co-ordinator were also heavy, which often meant that the cost was not a great deal less than a service provided by paid care attendants.

Host family schemes. Three services involving 'host families' were developed, which enabled carers to take a break of several days. Hosts were provided with expenses, rather than pay, but this could amount to a substantial amount per week. Although there was some success with these services, there were difficulties in finding host families with suitable accommodation, and sometimes resentment from carers that hosts were being paid for doing what the carer provided freely. There were also difficulties in placing people with severe disabilities, particularly since the host family houses had none of the aids and adaptations that made the caring task easier. This led two schemes for elderly people to experiment with placing volunteers in the disabled person's home for several days at a time: recruiting volunteers for this task was not easy, but some limited success was achieved.

Services for rural carers. Support for rural carers created particular difficulties because of scattered communities and transport problems, and frequently a lack of local voluntary organisations that were sufficiently robust to support any major new developments. However, projects were able to capitalise on the flexibility and overlapping responsibilities of rural services to piece together some interesting services using resources from a range of local agencies. (See Battle Carer Centre, and the account of rural work in East Sussex evaluation report (6)). The time scale for developing new services can be particularly slow in rural areas, and when allocating resources funders need to be aware of the additional costs required to cover the time taken by workers to travel to carers, or for the cost of transport for carers and their dependants.

For further information

1) An overview of schemes funded by the three consortia and some of the early lessons emerging: Dione Hills in collaboration with Sharon Haffenden, Tavistock Institute Working Paper, March 1988.

2) For an account of difficulties experienced by voluntary agencies running schemes and their staff; see 'Survey of employees from individual schemes', Paul Endersby and 'Enabling voluntary organisations to play a role in supporting carers in the community, some key issues', Jane Brotchie and Simon Northmore, in East Sussex Evaluation Report. Also the final research report from the Tavistock Institute.

3) Appendix A

4) Appendix B

5) Appendix C

6) Account of rural development work undertaken in East Sussex, in the East Sussex Evaluation Report.

4 CREATING CHANGE: THE ROLE OF CONSORTIA, GRANTS AND DEVELOPMENT WORKERS

As the main agency working on behalf of carers in their area, all three consortia interpreted the task of 'providing support' quite widely, and undertook both campaigning and development work in order to improve services and also to increase the recognition of carers' needs for services.

The main tools that they had to achieve change were:
1. the consortia themselves: these provided an important local forum bringing together influential members of voluntary and statutory organisations.
2. grant aid: to voluntary organisations to enable them to provide services to carers, and
3. development workers: staff appointed by the consortia.

Carer consortium as forum:

The consortia brought together representatives of key local voluntary organisations and statutory health and social services agencies. The balance of membership was different in each district: Stockport had a higher proportion of representatives from local voluntary agencies; Sandwell and East Sussex both had more representing local statutory organisations and national voluntary organisations. Full consortia meetings were held at least quarterly during the three years of the demonstration; sub committees met more frequently. Both gave members opportunities to find out about other agencies, to inform themselves about carer issues, and become involved in joint consideration of gaps in services in their area, and steps that might be taken to address these.

By the middle of the third year, most consortia members reported an increased understanding of carer issues both by themselves, and within the agencies they represented, as well as a general improvement in collaboration between their own agency and others working in the same field. Over a third reported their agencies undertaking joint work with other organisations in relation to carers. Nearly half thought that there had been a general improvement in attitude of statutory agencies towards the voluntary sector, promoted partly by the increased mutual understanding brought about by representatives from both working together on the consortia, and partly because the statutory agencies were impressed by consortia's abilities to distribute and evaluate grant aid (1).

Effecting change through grants:

The main way in which the consortia sought to change service provision for carers in their areas was through the distribution of grants. The availability of grants had clearly stimulated a number of local voluntary agencies to come up with a range of new services for carers (see section 3), although some had clearly taken the availability of funds as an opportunity to expand existing services directed at the disabled or ill person rather than services for the carer themselves. Although each consortium used the criteria for selection of schemes for grant aid as a way of influencing the kind of applications received, the ideas coming from local agencies fell short of covering the full range of possible services. For example, relatively few came up with ideas that catered for carers' needs for information and advice, and it was in this area that development workers had to intervene, to encourage local agencies to develop services in these areas, or to promote completely new organisations.

The importance of the role of grant aid was shown when consortia members completed a questionnaire on the outcome of the three year demonstration projects (1). On the whole, it was only members who represented agencies that received a grant who reported any new services for carers in their organisations, in spite of the general awareness of carers' needs most members reported within their organisations.

While most organisations were very committed to the services that they set up, the relatively high revenue expenditure required meant that they required substantial grants to cover running costs. As the end of the three years approached, the need to find local sources of funding for the new services put increasing pressure on the consortia to get carers onto local policy agendas. Statutory members of the consortia proved to be important links in this; even if they themselves were not in a position to influence funding policy, they were able to advise on how to approach those who were. Many different approaches were taken: seminars were set up to which senior managers and politicians were invited, individual approaches were made to councillors and senior managers, Joint Consultative Committees were lobbied, and various kinds of information material distributed: leaflets, articles, information packs, even a video (2). One measure of the success of the three consortia is the fact that the majority of projects that were still running at the end of the three years, obtained local funding to continue.

Development work undertaken by consortia staff:

Consortia varied in the amount of staff time and resources they allocated to general developmental activities (see section 2), but all undertook some activities designed to increase the awareness by public and professionals of the problems faced by carers. Action took place on both an individual and structural level (3). At an individual level, consortia staff provided training activities for health and social services staff (see section 5), produced information leaflets, and answered individual enquiries. They provided information and support to individuals in other local agencies who were setting up or running carer groups and services, and in East Sussex were themselves involved in setting up new carer support groups (3) (4).

At a structural level, they helped grant aided organisations through early difficulties, particularly organisational and managerial problems, and set up workshops at which these organisations could exchange ideas and experience. They helped establish new organisations in areas where there were few organisations in the voluntary sector that could run carer services (ie. in Sandwell and in rural areas in East Sussex (4)). Sometimes national or regional agencies were helped to set up branches in the areas, sometimes local individuals and professionals were located and helped to set up new local organisations. Sometimes staff were able to identify resources in local agencies which, although unable themselves to support new services, could offer premises or staff support to others. Many of the services established had their main costs covered by a grant from the consortium, but received some help from a number of other statutory and voluntary organisations (see tables in Appendices A, B and C).

Identifying the main areas in which action needed to be taken, and making contacts with people in the area who might be able to offer resources (if only the resource of their own time, as a committee member) was very time-consuming and results were frequently unpredictable. For some activities, development staff were inclined to provide a direct service: running a forum for local carer group organisers, or manning a carer information desk at a local social services team office. The difficulty with direct provision of this kind was that, if no one came forward to take over, the facility ended with the ending of the consortium funding. Those development projects that have continued after the end of the three year initiative have largely been those in which grants were awarded by the consortia so that local staff could be employed. In East Sussex, some activities have been taken over by a new 'Carer Council', established by the consortium towards the end of the DoH funding; resources for this have been found from local health authorities, social services (seconded staff) and trust funds. Although it was hoped that the carer resource centres would carry forward some of the developmental activities of the consortia in the three districts, their development work has on the whole been at a more local and practical level, and the difficulty in finding local funding for these has meant that their future has been insecure.

Consortia's contribution to change:

Overall, it is difficult at this stage to estimate the long term impact of the three consortia on services and provision for carers in their areas. Demonstration Districts were set up at a time when nationally, many changes were going on, or being contemplated, through changes in legislation and a number of other major initiatives for carers. Some of the activities that consortia undertook, such as trying to influence local professional and public attitudes to carers, cannot be seen in isolation from these wider developments. These activities were also inevitably long term, and it is too early to see their effects.

Nevertheless, in all three districts there is now a substantial increase in the number of services available in the voluntary sector and in two, at least, there continues to be voluntary organisation that brings together representatives of voluntary and statutory agencies to take an overview of carer services and promote carer issues in the area. How far the funding upon which these activities depend continues to be available from statutory sources, of course, remains to be seen: like most voluntary activity, funding is usually short term and vulnerable to changes in statutory policy.

Further information from:

1. Report on a questionnaire to consortium members: Tavistock Institute

Working paper, D. Hills, January 1989. Also reported in Final research report from the Institute.
2. Stockport Video 'Caring Together' (Crown Copyright) available from the DoH.
3. Final research report from the Tavistock Institute.
4. East Sussex Evaluation Report; particularly section on rural development work.

5 PROFESSIONALS AND CARERS

Although the carers interviewed in the Demonstration Districts project were all, by definition, in touch with a voluntary organisation, other research has shown that these are not the first place carers would look for support. Usually it is statutory services that are in touch with carers and in the position to refer them to services that can make their caring task easier. Within the Demonstration Districts, over 80% were in touch with at least one statutory service.

It was for this reason that all three consortia decided that raising awareness amongst professionals and statutory services was a vital part of their role, although their primary task was to improve support for carers through the voluntary sector. Difficulties with professionals and statutory services came up regularly in consultation meetings with carers in the early days of the programme. They also became apparent as new voluntary services were set up and were having difficulty in locating carers and getting referrals from professionals. Many professionals seemed unaware of what was going on in the voluntary sector, yet attempts to inform them were fraught with difficulties. Where providers of statutory services saw the needs of the disabled person as their primary responsibility, they often appeared to have little interest in services that would help carers.

Professionals' role in carer support:

In the survey of carers receiving services from the schemes (1), 80% of carers were in contact with their G.P., 63% received help from a nurse (district nurse or health visitor), 48% had seen a hospital consultant, and 44% a social worker. Between a quarter and a third received services such as respite care, aids and adaptations, meals on wheels, home helps, occupational therapists or physiotherapists. Although around half said that they had found their G.P., social worker or nurse 'very helpful', there was also criticism: around 10% found each of these 'not very helpful' with the number going up to 25% for occupational therapists or physiotherapists and to around 40% for meals on wheels, counsellors or psychologists, and community psychiatric nurses. Dissatisfaction may well have been due to the limited provision of these services, rather than the quality of the service itself. (1).

Interviews with carers (2) did indicate that the difficulties with statutory and professional services were often to do with limited resources, but carers also felt frustrated, and undervalued, when those attending their dependant ignored the importance of their own role in providing care and their difficulties with this role. They were particularly angry when they discovered that professionals had not informed them of services, or benefits, to which they were entitled, and which would have made the caring task a little easier.

Professionals, on the other side, are frequently stretched to capacity in dealing with the needs of people with disabilities or illness; carers are a background resource, probably noticed more when absent, or failing to provide care, than when they are caring. Many professionals themselves lack access to up-to-date information about relevant services or benefits; providing information of this kind was often not regarded as an important part of their job. Contact and co-operation between services, particularly where some are provided in the voluntary and some in the statutory sector, are often poor.

In workshops which brought together health care teams and carers (3), it became apparent that professional groups sometimes make unrealistic assumptions about the kind of support that is being provided by others. Social workers are seen to be the main providers of information on benefits and practical services, but only a minority of carers receive social worker support. Voluntary services are assumed to be providers of information, support, and sitting services although voluntary organisations know their role is quite low key. There are assumptions about the kind of support that should be provided by friends, neighbours and family members, although carers themselves often seem to expect little from neighbours and friends. Around 60% of carers using voluntary services said they received some help from family and friends, but dissatisfaction with help from this source was quite high (25% in one district) (4).

Strategies to increase professional awareness of carers:

Having identified that professionals were usually the people who had first contact with carers, all three districts took some steps to increase the level of understanding and information in statutory health and social services.

Local professionals and managers were invited to open meetings and seminars, and sent regular information about the activities being set up for carers. All three consortia also took steps to ensure that they had some representation in their membership from health authorities, social services departments, and G.P.s, the last of these being hardest to secure. In East Sussex, a training officer was recruited to provide information and training activities for professionals and in Stockport, the senior development officer undertook similar activities. In Sandwell, a representative from the social services was involved in the evaluation of schemes, in order to improve contact between social workers and the voluntary services for carers.

Training for staff in Health and Social Services:

It was not easy for consortia staff, being in the voluntary sector, to gain access to training activities in the statutory sector. Offers to provide an input about carers on existing courses were taken up by nursing services, and by social services departments, mostly for their home help and care staff; access to training for doctors was harder to gain. A variety of independent workshops were arranged for a mixture of professional groupings and levels. Different formats and locations were experimented with: busy professionals often found it hard to spare a full day; half day workshops were better attended, but it was difficult to cover all the material.

Feedback from participants (5) showed that the involvement of a carer in workshops was an important ingredient, their presence ensuring that all participants heard at first hand about the difficulties which carers experience. This seems to have more power to change established attitudes than theoretical or statistical presentations, or even role play. Videos were also helpful: these were available from the Department of Health and the King's Fund Informal Carers Unit. The Stockport consortium also made a video about some of the grant aided schemes and the carers using them, primarily to influence the councillors, but this also proved useful with professionals groups (6). Although many attending courses in East Sussex were already sympathetic to carer issues, they found the workshops helpful in confirming that they were working along the right lines. Some were already trying to change services in their own agencies; eg., one was trying to set up a link line for carers who ran into difficulties outside office hours, another was trying to get more respite beds in a local hospital.

General Practitioners and the Primary Health Care Team:

G.P.s did not usually attend these multi-disciplinary workshops. Both East Sussex and Stockport tried direct mailing of information, East Sussex producing a series of ten 'fact sheets' about carers similar to a series put out by the National Heart Association on heart disease. However, the response to questionnaires and invitations to contact the consortia for further information was poor (less than 2% in both districts), so it was difficult to assess how far information was read or found useful. Where feedback was received, it was apparent that G.P.s had shared the information with other professional members of the health care team, but not with receptionists.

In Stockport, health care teams felt that they wanted one telephone number, to which carers could be referred for information and advice, and leaflets advertising the availability of a telephone information line for carers were produced, particularly targetting receptionists and pharmacists. Fortunately the consortium had already funded a carers resource centre that provided such a help line: in many areas no such resource exists.

Although the local FPCs (now FHSAs) helped in the distribution of information to local G.P.s they do not have a direct role in training. However, in collaboration with the Royal College of General Practitioners, staff in East Sussex ran a series of workshops for primary health care teams (3 & 5). In these, team members identified a number of areas where improvements could be made: there could be a more co-ordinated response to families caring for handicapped members, ensuring that all professionals involved were kept informed of progress, that sufficient information was given to carers, and that visits by different professionals were staggered to ensure continuity of support. All workers involved with the situation needed to be alert to carers' needs, and the carers needed to be treated as members of the caring team with their own expertise and skill to contribute. While the need for key workers was recognised, it was frequently unclear who should be in this role; although G.P.s clearly had an important role, it is the nurse who has the regular day to day contact with the family, and nurses felt that they could take a large role in providing information and co-ordinating services, if the information and back up were available.

Overall, the three consortia showed that the deployment of relatively small levels of resources, particularly the time of specialist staff, could have an impact on increasing professional awareness of carers. Out of this, quite simple changes in procedure could bring considerable benefits to carers. However, to a large extent, the availability of this resource came to an end with the end of DoH funding and there was little evidence that the training role was picked up by other local organisations.

For further information

1. Report of Survey of Carers in East Sussex. Appendix B.
2. Final Research Report from the Tavistock Institute.
3. Caring for the Carers: report on multidisciplinary meetings in East Sussex; N. Channing Journal of Royal College of General Practitioners, March 1988.
4. Report of a survey of carers in Sandwell: Appendix C.
5. Report on the Training Work in East Sussex, East Sussex Evaluation Report.
6. Stockport video: Caring together (Crown Copyright) available from DoH.

6 EVALUATION OF SERVICES:

Evaluation of carer services funded by the three consortia was an important part of the Demonstration Districts programme and the methods adopted were to have an influence on the practice of other agencies in the three areas. The approach taken was developmental, contributing to the continuous learning process by all involved. With the support of the Tavistock research team, each consortium set up an evaluation procedure that fitted its own need for management information on the distribution of grants. Any monitoring system also needed to be flexible to fit in with the wide range of agencies grant aided; these varied from highly professional national voluntary agencies, to small local self-help groups. The services they provided were similarly varied.

Evaluation of grant aided services:

The approach adopted in each district was similar. Each grant aided scheme was required to give feed back on progress to their consortium through regular evaluation reports. The consortia gave broad guidelines as to the kind of information that was required, and included questions about process as well as outcomes, difficulties as well as successes. Early discussions were held with schemes individually about the kind of record keeping systems that might be required to assess progress towards their objectives, and the Tavistock researchers helped to run a workshop on evaluation in each district (1).

Consortia staff helped schemes to complete the reports, which provided an opportunity to jointly review any difficulties arising, and discuss ways of overcoming these at an early stage. Reports were then discussed by consortium members in their regular meetings, to which representatives of schemes were sometimes invited. This provided a useful way of keeping organisations represented on the consortia informed about overall progress, as well as utilising their advice on any problems arising. In Sandwell, social services staff took part in the evaluation procedure and the report was circulated widely in the borough; this provided an opportunity for different agencies to air their different expectations of the services grant aided.

Feedback from carers on their satisfaction with the services was handled differently. Following a series of in-depth interviews with carers by consortia staff and the Tavistock research team, (2), a questionnaire was designed and sent out, via the schemes, to carers receiving grant aided services in Sandwell and East Sussex. In Stockport, where one aim had been to prioritise the needs of carers looking after heavily dependent people, scheme organisers were asked to identify the numbers of clients with different kinds of dependency. Further interviews were carried out with a small sample of carers. (3,4,5).

An important feature of the evaluation process was that it allowed the recognition that different 'stake holders' might have differing expectations of carer support services, and that this affects the kind of evaluative questions asked. For example, most schemes started out with the explicit aim of providing help and support for carers and to meet their needs in a sensitive way; results from the carers questionnaire showed that most had been very successful in this. However, as organisations looked to local statutory sources for funding, questions began to be asked about how far services were enabling people to continue to be looked after in the community rather than in institutional care. These questions are hard to answer: so long as carers continue to provide care, it is difficult to establish whether they would do so without the service they are receiving. However, most schemes were able to point to a few carers where they felt that the situation would have been untenable or would have rapidly deteriorated without the service they were providing.

The other issue that came to prominence as other sources of funding were sought, was the relative cost and value for money for different kinds of services. Because of wide differences between projects, this was also difficult to answer: how can one compare a practical service such as sitting service, with one that provides information or a few hours of emotional support? While the feedback from carers indicated that many carers received information, advice and emotional support from practical services (which indicated that these were good value for money), this could only be sustained by allowing co-ordinators sufficient time and resources to undertake this work, and acknowledging that this was a central part of their workload. However, without an independent information and advice service, many carers would never have come to hear of the practical services. Information and advice services often picked up carers at an earlier stage in the caring situation – the importance of early advice compared to later support could only be determined through a longer term study.

In looking at the overall cost of services, it is important to recognise that most of the services set up were either fully staffed services, or ones in which a team of volunteers were supervised by paid staff. In practice, the savings through use of volunteers rather than paid staff were relatively small, and volunteers were less able to look after very disabled dependants. Although there were a number of very good schemes run entirely by volunteers, these were highly dependent on a few individuals with available time and commitment, and were consequently vulnerable to disruption if these were unable to continue.

There were other reasons why the 'value for money' questions were difficult to answer. In many of the schemes, the relatively low cost (see section 4), was partly due to subsidies they were receiving in kind from other services (eg accommodation). Sometimes the low cost was sustained because staff were on relatively low pay, and lacked support, training or pension rights. While this might have been sustainable in a short term and high profile project, the longer term effects of this might have been costly in high turnover or poor staff morale. On the other hand, the cost of some schemes appeared to be high because this initially included the cost of setting up a new organisation. This would probably have dropped as the service began to operate on a regular basis.

Evaluation of development work:

Evaluation of the developmental activities of the consortia was particularly difficult to achieve. In a time limited project it is only possible to demonstrate interim measures of success: services or groups were established, but how far permanent changes were achieved in services or attitudes can be hard to demonstrate. Several of the development staff were interviewed individually and most of these were able to report a number of notable achievements. Consortium members, who were representative of other local agencies, reported their appreciation of the work undertaken in the support of new services, provision of training, and general campaigning work undertaken on behalf of carers. The fact that all continuing schemes were able to obtain further funding from local sources, in spite of a hostile funding environment, is no small measure of the success of the campaigning work undertaken, although other moves to enhance the status of carers nationally were clearly also having their effect in the three districts as well.

Two important points emerged from the evaluation of development work. One was that projects that depended upon the input of the development workers themselves were less likely to be sustained after the worker left, than those in which an independent management group was established and funding obtained for a local worker. (See Section 5). This is important to note because independent projects can take longer to set up than those directly provided.

The other point was that the management and support of the development workers posed a difficulty for nearly all the voluntary committees, leading to lost work time through lack of direction, unclarity of role, or loss of morale because expectations were unrealistic. In some cases the difficulty was that management was undertaken by new committees which were themselves unclear or disunited about what they hoped to achieve. Research into the needs of the area prior to the setting the job description, and provision of an experienced supervisor or advisor, made the task of the worker easier (2 and 6).

Additional information from:

1. Evaluation as a development activity: Dione Hills and Sharon Haffenden. Paper in 'Evaluation support for carers' conference report. SPRU 1987
2. Final Research report from the Tavistock Institute
3. Caring together in Stockport: final report. Appendix A
4. Report on a Survey of Carers in East Sussex. Appendix B
5. Report on a Survey of Carers in Sandwell. Appendix C
6. East Sussex Evaluation Report.

Appendix A

CARING TOGETHER IN STOCKPORT
FINAL REPORT MARCH 1989
Sharon Haffenden

CONTENTS

CARING TOGETHER IN STOCKPORT

Final Report – March 1989

1. Background

1.1 In 1984, the Secretary of State for Health announced a £10.5 million programme, *Helping the Community to Care*. The aim of the three year programme was to help volunteers, families and others to care for those who need support, and it illustrated the concern of Ministers at that time to promote community care.

1.2 One element of the programme, was the establishment of three Demonstration Districts, whose broad purpose was to focus on carers across the whole spectrum of age and disability, and to develop voluntary sector services to meet their needs, while also raising the profile of carers with both service providers and funders of the service. The three Districts were in Stockport, East Sussex and Sandwell.

1.3 A new aspect of the Demonstration Districts was the use of local voluntary sector consortia to distribute the funds available. The £600,000 made available to each District was seen as 'pump-priming' money and therefore given only on a three year time-limited basis. The Department of Health envisaged that the Demonstration Districts should be a partnership between the voluntary and statutory sectors, and this proved to be the case, anticipating the new working relationships proposed by Sir Roy Griffiths. Full details of the different models of local collaboration are given in a *Report of a DHSS Seminar on the three Demonstration Districts for Voluntary Sector Carer Support held at Aston University* (1).

1.4 The original aims of the three Demonstration Districts were:

(1) Edited by Sharon Haffenden, 1988, available from Department of Health

(i) to enhance developments and promote new initiatives in the voluntary sector in supporting informal carers in specific local authority areas, in order to demonstrate the value of these

(ii) to provide reports for use in other areas to promote support for informal carers and engage with other developments on a wide front

(iii) to monitor and identify outcomes and indicators for the future in terms of support for carers.

1.5 In Stockport, the Consortium of voluntary organisations was known as *Caring Together in Stockport*, and established a frame work for the project:

(i) development of schemes

(ii) monitoring and evaluation of schemes

(iii) dissemination of lessons learned.

The DoH sponsored the Tavistock Institute to lead the monitoring and evaluation of the three Demonstration Districts, and to lead a dissemination phase (2).

1.6 Over twenty schemes were funded over the three years in Stockport, including some one-off activities such as consultation meetings with carers. This final report gives details of the final evaluation of the twelve ongoing schemes in Stockport.

2. Introduction

2.1 Included in this report are the twelve current Caring Together schemes, funded during the period 1986-1988, with monies from the DHSS "Helping the Community to Care" programme. Details of the schemes are shown in Table 1.

2.2 The Caring Together Consortium had agreed that their own local evaluation should try to ascertain whether their initial goals in funding individual schemes had been effectively achieved; whether

(2) Demonstration Districts Final Report by Dione Hills, available from the Tavistock Institute of Human Relations.

the schemes had been targeted on those carers looking after the more dependent people and whether the situation of carers in Stockport had improved since the Consortium-funded schemes began.

2.3 The sources for the following information are the schemes themselves. Interviews with a small number of carers in Stockport are the subject of a separate report (3).

2.4 Appended to this report is a summary of factors affecting the development of four schemes, started under the Demonstration District but not continued.

Table 1. *Details of schemes and their costs*

Scheme	Grant given £	Use of Volunteers	Other non-cash Subsidies
1. Offerton Neighbourhood Care – recruits, trains, supports and places volunteers to assist carers in a local neighbourhood with practical help	6,200	Paid organiser only (P/T) + 30 volunteers	Health Authority accommodation, Local Authority payroll, CVS supervision
2. Cancer Aid & Listening Line for carers in Stockport – recruits, trains, supports and places volunteers to assist carers of cancer sufferers	14,800	Paid organiser (32 hrs) & P/T clerical help + 25 volunteers	LA accommodation, clerical help
3. Boys & Girls Welfare Society Linkways – Leisure, social and befriending scheme for young people, (16-30) with physical disability, by recruiting volunteers	15,000	Paid (F/T) organiser only + 21 volunteers	BGWS accommodation, supervision and payroll
4. Pines Holiday/Respite Home; Activities & Leisure Scheme – recruiting volunteers to befriend Pines users (young people & children with learning difficulties) to enable them to engage in additional activities in and out of The Pines	9,000	(F/T) paid organiser + 20 volunteers.	Pines accommodation, + supervision. LA payroll

(3) Carer Support Profiles – Lucette Tucker; available from Sharon Haffenden, 3 Towncroft Lane, Bolton BL1 5EW.

Table 1. *Details of schemes and their costs* (Cont'd)

Scheme	Grant given £	Use of Volunteers	Other non-cash Subsidies
5. Stockport Day Centre for Recovering mentally ill – extension of hours for Sunday & evening opening	13,000	No volunteers Paid F/T post	LA/HA accommodation LA payroll SDC supervision
6. Citizens Advice Bureau Home Visiting Service – CAB advice to carers in their own home	10,000	No volunteers Paid P/T post	CAB accommodation; supervision; LA payroll
7. Signpost Resource Centre – information; carers' groups – for all Stockport carers	45,000	5 paid staff (1 F/T + 4 P/T) plus 4 volunteers	LA accommodation + payroll
8. Crossroads Care Attendant Scheme provides practical help and respite for carers of people with physical and/or mental handicap (under 65)	25,000	All paid staff (1 P/T Asst organiser + care attendants) No volunteers	LA accommodation payroll, Crossroads supervision
9. Age Concern Stockport Day Sitting Service – provides respite and practical help for carers of elderly people, especially confused elderly	25,000	All paid staff 1 P/T organiser + care attendants. No volunteers	LA accommodation + payroll, ACS supervision
10. Charnwood Day Nursery Family Support Worker – advice and support to to special needs children and their families at the day nursery (under 5's)	7,500	1 Paid P/T staff No volunteers	Charnwood supervision, payroll, accommodation
11. North West Fellowship Family Support Worker – advice and support to carers of schizophrenia sufferers plus befriending for sufferers	14,000	No volunteers 1 paid F/T staff	NWF supervision LA accommodation and payroll
12. COMBAT Huntington's Chorea – Relaxation & stress management, and social work assistance for carers of Huntington's Chorea sufferers	7,335	No volunteers 1 paid P/T staff	COMBAT payroll and supervision

3. The evaluation

Table 2. *Numbers of carers benefiting from the schemes*

Scheme	Total Carers who have used the scheme (1)	Carers benefiting monthly (2)	
		Carers	Cared for (3)
Offerton Neighbourhood Care	250	15	—
CALL Carers	168	20	—
BGWS Linkways	41	(20)	20
Pines Leisure	100	(35)	35
Stockport Day Centre (Extended Hours)	42	(15)	15 (3)
CAB Home Visitor	300	15	—
Signpost Resource Centre	530	42	—
Crossroads	132	45	—
Age Concern Stockport Day Sitting Service	200	36	—
Charnwood Family Support Worker	70	47	—
NWF Family Support Worker	42	28	—
COMBAT Relaxation/SW	17	15	—
TOTAL	1892	333	

Notes

1. Ie since its inception; Offerton Care Scheme November 1986; CALL Carers November 1987; BGWS January 1988; PALS August 1986; Stockport D.C. November 1986; CAB HVS January 1987; Signpost March 1987; Crossroads May 1986; ACS Day Sitting August 1986; Charnwood FSW January 1987; NWF January 1988; COMBAT September 1987.

2. The distinction is that three schemes (BGWS, PALS, Stockport DC) are specifically focused on the cared for, and have minimal contact with carers. The carers benefiting figure is bracketed to indicate that they benefit indirectly.

3. There are special problems in getting accurate information on the carers of users of Stockport Day Centre. This average is based on two sessions only.

Table 3. *The level and nature of the service provided to carers*

Scheme	Service to Carers Monthly Average	Nature of Service
Offerton Neighbourhood Care	4 hours	Practical help and emotional support
CALL Carers	15-20 hours	(as above)
BGWS Linkways (See Note 1)	(12-15 hours)	Enhancing independence of users. Carers get respite indirectly; also hope & emotional support
Pines Leisure Scheme	(12 hours)	Enhancing independence of users. Carers get respite indirectly; also hope for the future
Stockport Day Centre (Extended Hours)	(N/A)	Drop in Centre and activities for users. Indirectly carers are getting respite
CAB Home Visitor	4 hours	Telephone or domiciliary CAB advice
Signpost Resource Centre	10/15 mins	Support and information, development work
Crossroads	12 hours	Practical help and respite
Age Concern Day Sitting	12-15 hours	(as above)
Charnwood Family Support Worker	5 hours	Liaison & advocacy with statutory bodies. Advice, emotional support, limited practical help eg transport.
Northwest Fellowship Family Support Worker	2 hours	Liaison & advocacy with statutory bodies. Befriending for sufferer. Advice, emotional support, limited practical help, eg transport.
COMBAT Relaxation/ Social Work	4.5 hours	Relaxation therapy, specialist advice, emotional support, carers group, limited practical help, eg transport.

Notes

1. Bracketed figures indicate that the direct recipient of help is the cared for person.

Table 4. *What do carers like best about the schemes?*

Offerton Neighbourhood Care – carers in all situations; many carers over 60	Being able to telephone for "one off" help when they feel low; the offer of practical support "and not just someone who goes in and preaches"; "I feel someone at last is going to do something to help and not just talk about it".
CALL Carers – carers of cancer sufferers	The volunteers are people who have been in the situation themselves, and have more time for them than professionals.
BGWS Linkways – carers of young adults with physical disability	They feel encouraged to see their child going out with other young people. Parents get some respite, also are emotionally relieved to see their child developing a social network outside the family.
Pines – carers of young people and children with severe learning difficulties	The fact that their child receives more stimulation by having their individual needs and interests met; also that their child takes part in non-segregated activities.
Stockport Day Centre – Extended Hours – carers of people recovering from mental illness	Availability and informality of the Centre; also it is the only resource available at weekends/ evenings for the recovering mentally ill.
CAB Home Visitor – carers in all situations	The quick and efficient home visiting service; the home visiting officer is seen as an ally and advocate.
Signpost Resource Centre – carers in all situations	The organisation is providing a service particularly for them; *one* telephone call can put them in touch with services and support.
Crossroads – carers of adults & children with physical/mental mental disabilities	The flexibility – service is arranged to suit the carer, and might change every week; also the practical help is geared to their own pace.
Age Concern Day Sitting – carers of elderly people	(i) It is the only service to this group of carers that meets their needs as well as the needs of the person cared for (ii) the informal approach (iii) flexibility (iv) home-based service (v) free service (vi) peace of mind.
Charnwood Family Support Worker – carers of under-fives with special needs	That the FSW has *time* to listen, advise and provide practical support focused on the carer not the child; also the help is available in evenings, weekends, and school holidays. Some carers feel that the non-statutory FSW is less threatening than other professionals.

These comments are summaries of written and verbal feedback from carers to schemes.

Table 4. *What do carers like best about the schemes?* (Cont'd)

North West Fellowship Family Support Worker – carers of schizophrenia sufferers	(i) Having *one* person to contact in a crisis, (ii) early intervention when problems arise, (iii) consistent personal contact (with carer and sufferer), (iv) liaison and advocacy with professionals.
COMBAT (Huntington's Chorea) Relaxation/Social Work – carers of HC sufferers	Regular availability; frequent and consistent personal contact; specialist knowledge of the condition; has helped to give carers more confidence in themselves and their ability to cope.

These comments are summaries of written and verbal feedback from carers to schemes.

Table 5. *Outstanding concerns raised by schemes on behalf of carers*

Offerton Neighbourhood Care (all types of carers, including elderly carers)	• continued information required • emotional support & reassurance required.
BGWS Linkways (carers of young people with physical disabilities)	• parents can be reluctant to allow the young people to have financial independence using the allowances intended for them.
Pines Leisure Scheme (carers of young people with severe learning difficulties)	• parents still accept segregation of their children.
CAB Home Visitor (carers in all situations)	• carers dissatisfied with the help from statutory services and lack of consultation with professionals.
Signpost Resource Centre (carers in all situations)	• continued stress and isolation for carers • local service in neighbourhoods to enable personal contacts to develop.
Crossroads (carers of people under 65)	• inadequate day centre provision for people with physical handicaps.
Age Concern Stockport Day Sitting (carers of people over 65)	• continuity of care attendant enables carer to use c.a. as sympathetic confidante.
Charnwood Family Support Worker (carers of under 5's with special needs)	• getting aids and adaptations is made difficult and over-long by procedural complexities and organisational boundaries. • statementing of children with special needs has not been effectively done, resulting in the recent establishment of a parents' support group for paramedical help in schools.
North West Fellowship Family Support Worker (carers of schizophrenia sufferers)	• difficulty in gaining hospital admission and services *prior* to breakdown. • lack of support in day to day management of the sufferer at home.

Table 6. *Proportion of cared for who require considerable care*

(i) Activities of Daily Living Capacity

Dependency Scheme	Level 1 (See note 1)	Level 2 (See note 2)	Total
Offerton Neighbourhood Care	0%	14%	14%
CALL Carers	17%	13%	30%
BGWS Linkways	13%	47%	60%
Pines Leisure	34%	40%	74%
Stockport Day Centre (Extended Hours)	N/A	N/A	N/A
CAB Home Visitor	33%	27%	60%
Signpost Resource Centre	—	27%	27% See Note 3
Crossroads	76%	24%	100% See Note 4
Age Concern Stockport Day Sitting	35%	50%	85%
Charnwood Family Support	36%	34%	70%
NWF Family Support	0%	0%	0%
COMBAT Relaxation/SW	5%	90%	95%

Notes

SOURCE OF DEPENDENCY SCALES: Pfeiffer scales, designed by Duke Longitudinal Study in Aging, U.S.A.

1. Level 1 ie the cared for have *completely impaired activities of daily living capacity* ie they need help throughout day and/or night to cope with personal care. Requiring very frequent supervision (once every two or three hours).
2. Level 2 ie the cared for have *severely impaired ADL capacity* ie they need daily help with personal care.
3. Signpost do not make home visits, and cannot therefore assess this on the basis of telephone information.
4. 20% are children.

(ii) Severe Physical Health problems

Health Scheme	Level 1 (Note 1)	Level 2 (Note 2)	Total
Offerton Neighbourhood Care	Nil	14%	14%
CALL Carers	31%	37%	68%

Table 6. *Proportion of cared for who require considerable care* (Cont'd)

(ii) Severe Physical Health problems (Cont'd)

Health Scheme	Level 1 (Note 1)	Level 2 (Note 2)	Total
BGWS Linkways	Nil	Nil	Nil
Pines Leisure	Nil	Nil	Nil
Stockport Day Centre (Extended Hours)	N/A	N/A	N/A
CAB Home Visitor	13%	7%	20%
Signpost Resource Centre	—	5%	5% See Note 3
Crossroads	14%	86%	100%
Age Concern Stockport Day Sitting	30%	55%	85%
Charnwood Family Support	Nil	40%	40%
NWF Family Support	0%	0%	0%
COMBAT Relaxation/SW	—	100%	100%

Notes

1. Level 1 ie the cared for have *totally impaired physical health* ie confined to bed and requiring full-time medical assistance or nursing care to maintain bodily functions.

2. Level 2 ie the cared for have one or more illnesses or disabilities which are either severely painful or life threatening, or which require extensive medical treatment.

3. As indicated above, Signpost are unable to make this assessment.

(iii) Severe Mental Health Problems

Mental Health Scheme	Level 1 (Note 1)	Level 2 (Note 2)	Total
Offerton Neighbourhood Care	Nil	Nil	Nil
CALL Carers	Nil	17%	17%
BGWS Linkways	Nil	Nil	Nil
Pines Leisure	Nil	34%	34% Note 3
Stockport Day Centre (Extended Hours)	10%	Nil	10% Note 4
CAB Home Visitor	Nil	Nil	Nil Note 5

Table 6. *Proportion of cared for who require considerable care* (Cont'd)

(iii) Severe Mental Health Problems (Cont'd)

Scheme / Mental Health	Level 1 (Note 1)	Level 2 (Note 2)	Total	
Signpost Resource Centre	—	—	—	Note 6
Crossroads	22%	Nil	22%	
Age Concern Stockport Day Sitting	35%	50%	85%	
Charnwood Family Support	N/A	N/A	N/A	Note 7
NWF Family Support	13%	25%	38%	Note 8
COMBAT Relaxation/SW	5%	95%	100%	

Notes

1. Level 1 ie *completely impaired mental health* ie has grossly psychotic symptoms or is completely impaired intellectually, and requires either intermittent or constant supervision because of clearly abnormal or potentially harmful behaviour.

2. Level 2 ie *severely impaired mental health* ie has severe psychiatric symptoms and/or severe intellectual impairment, which interfere with routine judgements and decision-making in every day life.

3. P.A.L.S. – A further 26% of those care for in this month had mildly impaired mental health.

4. Stockport Day Centres figures may seem low; the Centre deals only with the recovering mentally ill.

5. CAB – This breakdown is based on November; however usually about 10% of carers are looking after people with Alzheimer's Disease.

6. As above, Signpost is unable to assess this.

7. Charnwood – not applicable as carers are looking after children under 5.

8. The majority of carers supported by the NWF FSW are looking after (Level 3) sufferers with moderately impaired mental health (34%), and a further 28% look after those with mildly impaired mental health (Level 4).

Table 7. *Carers in poor physical/mental health*

	Carers' Health					
	Physical Health (1)			Mental Health (1)		
Scheme	Level 2	Level 3	Level 4	Level 2	Level 3	Level 4
Offerton Neighbourhood Care	14%	7%	14%	Nil	Nil	Nil
CALL Carers	3%	5%	25%	Nil	Nil	4%
BGWS Linkways	Nil	Nil	Nil	Nil	Nil	Nil
Pines Leisure	8%	Nil	Nil	Nil	Nil	Nil
Stockport Day Centre (Extended Hours)	N/A	N/A	N/A	N/A	N/A	N/A Note 2
CAB Home Visitor	Nil	7%	7%	Nil	Nil	Nil
Signpost Resource Centre	N/A	N/A	N/A	—	—	15% Note 3
Crossroads	8%	4%	18%	Nil	Nil	Nil
Age Concern Stockport Day Sitting	10%	20%	10	Nil	20%	10%
Charnwood Family Support	6%	Nil	Nil	Nil	Nil	8%
NWF Family Support	3%	6%	6%	0%	0%	13%
COMBAT Relaxation/SW	Nil	Nil	30%	Nil	15%	25%

Notes

1. The Level 1 classifications of physical and mental health impairment, given above, are not applicable here.

   Level 2 physical and mental health classifications – described in Table 3 (ii) and (iii) above.

   Level 3 physical health classification ie has one or more diseases or disabilities which are either painful or which require substantial medical treatment.

   Level 4 physical health ie has minor illness and/or disabilities which might benefit from medical treatment.

   Level 3 mental health ie has definite psychiatric symptoms and/or moderate intellectual impairment.

   Level 4 mental health ie has mild psychiatric symptoms and/or mild intellectual impairment.

Notes (Cont'd)

2. Stockport Day Centre has minimal contact with carers, so this information is not available.

3. Signpost Stockport were also unable to collect this information.

NB: Most schemes do not routinely collect this information. *The figures here substantially underestimate the incidence of poor physical and mental health, and other problems particularly stress and exhaustion.*

Table 8. *Older Carers*

	Carers
Schemes	% over 60
Offerton Neighbourhood Care	50
CALL Carers	27
BGWS Linkways	10
Pines Leisure	18
Stockport Day Centre	40
CAB Home Visitor	40
Signpost Resource	49
Crossroads	40
Age Concern Day Sitting	33
Charnwood Family Support	0
NWF Family Support	53
COMBAT Relaxation/SW	33

Note

BGWS Linksways and P.A.L.S. are aimed at younger cared for persons. Charnwood is only for under-fives and their families.

Table 9. *Demand for the Service*

Scheme	Indicators of Demand
Offerton Neighbourhood Care	All demands are met
CALL Carers	All demands have been met except for some requests for transport; but volunteers are not being replaced/retrained while long term funding is uncertain.

Table 9. *Demand for the Service* (Cont'd)

Scheme	Indicators of Demand
BGWS Linkways	Waiting list of approx. 10, at all times
Pines Leisure Scheme	All cared for persons able to use the scheme (76) are matched, but ideally the service should have 76 volunteers to enable the person cared for to use the scheme more frequently and flexibly.
Stockport Day Centre (Extended Hours)	Anyone attending the centre is accommodated, but only by increasing pressure on staff. Two part-time staff are available to cover the extended hours, which may result in a ratio of one staff to sixteen users.
CAB Home Visitor	The HV Officer, a part-time post (25 hrs) is only able to respond to carers' requests for a home visit after a wait of approximately one week. Though the numbers of new referrals fluctuates, there are a number of carers who use the service on a regular basis.
Signpost Resource Centre	No waiting list. All referrals followed up within 24 hours. But service is still reaching a very small proportion (2%) of carers in Stockport
Crossroads	The number of requests for additional help exceed the amount of hours of care available.
Age Concern Day Sitting	Small waiting list (currently 13); many carers would like extra hours.
Charnwood Family Support Worker	The FSW and nursery staff try to meet the needs of all who seek their help.
NWF Family Support Worker	All requests for help are attended to.
COMBAT Relaxation/SW	The demand from this small but pressured group of carers requires a full-time worker for emotional support, psycho-sexual counselling, stress management and specialist advice on Huntington's Chorea.

4. Final comments on schemes

4.1 *How effective are the schemes in targeting carers?*

4.1.1 This final report is on the twelve ongoing Caring Together schemes, which collectively have been used by approximately 1,892 ie 6% of the total population of carers in Stockport (estim. 30,000). Carers are a neglected group, but also they are a difficult group to reach, and caring covers a wide spectrum, so it is not straightforward making a judgement on this figure. The Caring Together consortium tried to target those carers looking after the most dependent people, particularly by grant-aiding Age Concern Stockport Day Sitting Service (caring for a confused or demented elderly person is a huge burden), Crossroads, Cancer Aid & Listening Line for Carers, Pines Leisure Scheme, Stockport Day Centre and North West Fellowship Family Support Worker (carers of mental illness sufferers feel they have special problems) and COMBAT (Huntington's Chorea is very stressful on the carer, physically and mentally). Extrapolating from research done elsewhere in the country (4) there are an estimated 22% (5,400) of carers in Stockport who are looking after people who need help with all personal care tasks, including feeding. Only Crossroads reports that 100% of its users ie carers, are looking after people (including children) with completely or severely impaired Activities for Daily Living Capacity. Two other schemes, COMBAT's Relaxation/Social Work Support and Age Concern's Day Sitting Service also report that high proportions, 95% and 85% respectively, of their carers are in this position. One hundred percent of the carers supported by COMBAT care for people who have severely or completely impaired physical *and* mental health. Crossroads reports that 100% of its users care for people with completely or severely impaired physical health. Eighty five percent of Age Concern's users also care for people with completely or severely impaired physical health. *There can be no doubt that, in Stockport, Crossroads, Age Concern and COMBAT are targeted on those carers in most need of support*. They provide an intensive service (Crossroads and Age Concern clients could expect 12 hours of service in a month and COMBAT's clients get four and a half hours per month). Age Concern and Crossroads concentrate on providing respite and practical help, while the COMBAT worker provides emotional support, help with psychosexual problems, stress management and limited practical help, eg transport. This part-time worker is concentrating on a small group of 15 carers each month, while Age Concern and Crossroads, with their staff of paid care-attendants help 36 and 45 carers respectively each month. Other schemes that are also targeted on those carers looking after people who require considerable care are The Pines Volunteers Leisure Scheme and Charnwood Day Nursery Family Support Worker, Cancer Aid & Listening Line volunteers and North West Fellowship

(4) *Who Cares in Southwark*, 1984, Sharon Bonny (Carers' National Association)

Family Support Worker. *This would indicate that the Consortium aim to target those carers looking after the most dependent people has been met to a significant degree by these seven schemes.*

4.1.2 Carers' need for support cannot always be judged by the problems of the person they look after. *Age Concern Stockport Day Sitting Service and COMBAT report the largest proportion of carers who themselves have impaired physical and/or mental health* (Table 7). CALL Carers Stockport and Offerton Neighbourhood Care report the highest incidence of poor physical health among the carers, 33% and 35% respectively. Two other schemes, Crossroads and North West Fellowship report over a quarter of carers having impaired physical and/or mental health (Table 7). Other problems, such as exhaustion and stress, were not specifically measured in this evaluation, but have been reported by at least five schemes. The Offerton Neighbourhood Care Scheme's reporting of poor physical health problems may be correlated to it having a large proportion (50%) of carers over 60 amongst the schemes. NWF had the highest proportion of carers over 60 (53%) and four other schemes reported 40% or more over 60 (Table 8).

4.2 *Have the schemes addressed the needs of carers?*

4.2.1 *All* the schemes consider they have been effective in meeting those needs that they had set out to relieve. Most report that they provide other help, particularly information and emotional support, perhaps because a gap exists which no-one has proper responsibility to fill, or because carers often develop personal relationships with staff or volunteers, and prefer to ask them rather than battle their way through a large and complex system. Four schemes were praised by carers for their friendly advice and support in interviews, specifically Offerton Neighbourhood Care Scheme, The Pines Respite Home itself, COMBAT and Crossroads.

4.2.2 Also, some quantitative measure of the schemes are shown in Table 3. Among volunteer schemes, CALL Carers, Pines Leisure Scheme and Linkways volunteers have the highest level of service to carers. Among paid schemes, Crossroads and Age Concern, are highest (12-15 hrs). It is worth noting that CALL's carers are getting the same monthly average level of input from volunteers as Crossroads and Age Concern's carers get from a paid service (Table 3) but the level of dependency of the person cared for is much greater in the two paid schemes. Of the two schemes providing information and advice, the CAB Home Visitor means that where necessary, a carer can receive a more intense level of support as required, complementing the faster through-put of Signpost Resource Centre.

4.2.3 Stockport Day Centre (for recovering mentally ill), like the Pines Leisure Scheme and Linkways, is a service focused on the person cared for. Carers are rarely seen at the Centre, though a census indicated that of 31 centre users, 24 had weekly or more frequent contact with their carer, although only 3 of the 31 actually lived with the carer. In these circumstances, it is hard to know whether carers actually perceive a benefit of respite or whether the Centre's extended opening hours gives them just a sense of relief, because *it is there*. Organisers of the Pines and Linkways schemes try to see carers from time to time, and have received positive feedback (Table 4).

4.3 *Feedback from carers*

4.3.1 All schemes report that they receive positive feedback from carers in informal ways eg conversations, and letters. Feedback shown in Table 4, ranges from carers liking the flexibility and the quick service, to being very pleased to see independence encouraged in their young son or daughter, which has started to break the mould of existing services in a positive way. However, it is clear from experience here and elsewhere that carers' demands are modest and they are grateful for the personal interest and individual attention that they receive from the voluntary sector schemes. It is interesting to hear carers say they appreciate having something *specially for them*. They also like the non-threatening status of non-statutory organisations (eg Charnwood, a voluntary sector run day nursery).

4.3.2 Organisers do hear concerns from the carers too (see Table 5). Briefly, they report there is still a need for *more* day time opportunities for young people with physical handicaps, freely available drop-in facilities for carers, *more* practical help, *more* emotional support, and a more sympathetic service from the statutory sector.

4.4 *Conclusions*

4.4.1 The Caring Together schemes in this report are only reaching a small percentage of carers in Stockport, but a significant proportion are those who are in greatest need of support because they are looking after highly dependent people. Crossroads, Age Concern Stockport and COMBAT emerge strongly, but then they were three schemes that were consolidating and extending their existing work. Some of the other organisations have pioneered new services, and Signpost has the added disadvantage of starting up as a new organisation, though given time, it may make more impact. Other schemes, for example, Linkways, Cancer Aid & Listening Line, Stockport Day centre, CAB Home Visitor, Crossroads, Age Concern Stockport and the three Family Support Workers – Charnwood, North West Fellowship and COMBAT, are all working at full stretch, and can only accommodate more carers by reducing the quality or quantity of service to existing users, and by putting more pressure on individual staff.

4.4.2 Three of the schemes are focused on the person cared for. It is interesting to note that in two cases (Linkways and the Pines Leisure Scheme), parents were beginning to report benefits for *themselves*, through their children participating in non-segregated, independence-orientated schemes. The Day Centre might benefit from closer communication with carers, though there are special difficulties with this, because of the feelings of the users of the Centre.

4.4.3 *These schemes have done much to improve the situation for carers in Stockport, providing information and advice, practical help in the home, regular respite and emotional support for carers*. The Consortium has demonstrated that the non-statutory sector is valued by carers because it is able to offer help on a more personal basis. Emotional support comes naturally when trust has developed, and this is more feasible when there is continuity in personal contacts. Practical help and respite offered by the non-statutory sector is valued by carers because it is tailored to individual circumstances as far as possible, and because it recognises the contribution of the carer, and tries to replicate it rather than change it.

4.4.4 The Consortium has demonstrated also that volunteers can make a significant contribution – one third of the schemes depend on volunteers, but the provision of the regular respite and help with caring tasks that carers rely on, can only be provided through a paid service.

4.4.5 The situation for carers in Stockport is changing through a number of influences, national and local. Locally, the Demonstration District has been the catalyst not only for service development but for a new awareness of the carers' perspective.

Appendix A1

Summary of evaluation of three schemes not funded for 1988/89

1. Introduction

1.1 This appendix is a summary of the final evaluation of three schemes which were not funded for 1988/89, but ran from 1986 to March 1988. This summary is also based on the same questions that have been posed to ongoing schemes, ie whether the scheme was of benefit to carers, and whether or not organisational or external factors prevented the scheme from making the progress expected.

2. Were the schemes of benefit to the carers?

2.1 The need for all three schemes had been demonstrated – two by research findings (one was local scientific research) and one by discussions with professionals and carers.

2.2 Demand for the schemes did not emerge however – two schemes were not used by carers, but the third showed signs that it would have been, if organisational and external factors had not held it back. The demand for the first two schemes might have increased, if the organisational issues had been addressed promptly.

3. Organisational and external factors

3.1 It was a combination of external and organisational factors that hindered the schemes from making progress. It is important to point out that similar problems that afflicted these three schemes, also affected schemes in the other two Demonstration Districts.

3.2 Organisational factors:

(i) Management Committees – in two schemes, the committee members were unclear about their role, and so did not give the staff the support and direction they required.

In one of these, the staff member found it difficult to report to a committee after being used to working alone. However, one criterion of the DoH funding was that grants could only be made to formally-constituted organisations.

(ii) "Too much too soon" – one organisation was entirely new, and its difficulties arose because the staff member concerned was trying to run the new scheme as a paid employee, while at the same time running a separate long-established scheme as an independent volunteer. One other organisation was relatively new (less than three years old), and never seriously took on board the aims of the funding it had applied for. The third scheme was set up by a longer-established organisation, which had not considered the implications of the new service for their existing service. The latter two organisations were local and independent, while the third one had a very loose and fairly unsupportive relationship with a national organisation.

(iii) Lack of clarity of role and task of new workers – this was a problem in one scheme, where a new worker with a specific task was absorbed into an existing staff team and expected to also share their tasks.

(iv) Lack of flexibility – all three schemes showed this – having fixed upon a model for the scheme, they determinedly set about implementing it, even though in two schemes it was not proving successful with carers; in the third scheme, lack of flexibility hindered recruitment of "substitute carers".

(v) Finding carers – this was a problem for two schemes; however, it was these two schemes that did not adapt the model – another model might have attracted more carers in both cases.

3.3 External factors:

(i) Social Security changes in Regulations governing payment of allowances – this hampered one scheme for nine months, as the DSS failed to clarify the position.

Lack of referrals from statutory sector staff – this affected two schemes, even though one of them had had "a presence" in the field for some time, and was set up against a background of scientific and social research evidence.

4. Conclusion

4.1 Knowing that there is a need for a scheme is not enough. Time must be allowed to plan and set up the scheme, and to consider the implications of the new service for the existing organisation, *prior* to the delivery of the service to carers. Time must also be allowed for a scheme to gain credibility with both carers and professionals, especially when an organisation is new.

4.2 Voluntary Organisations should be more prepared to take advice. This is readily available from umbrella organisations (eg GMCVS, NCVO, Volunteer Centre) as well as in books and other literature. All three of these organisations had not fully explored the implications of their new work for carers adequately at the outset, and when problems arose two schemes were reluctant to take advice on the way through them.

Appendix B

CARER STRESS AND CARER SUPPORT
Report of a survey of carers using schemes in East Sussex

Wendy Wallace

CONTENTS

This report is a slightly abbreviated version of a chapter in the East Sussex final evaluation report. Appendix 1 has been added in order to present information on schemes, for comparative purposes, in the same format as has been used in the reports from the other two districts.

1 Introduction

In 1988 the Office of Population Censuses and Surveys report based on the 1985 General Household Survey indicated an estimated six million carers in Great Britain, some 14% of the adult population. On the basis of the most recent estimate of the adult population of East Sussex (OPCS 1987) there are upwards of 78,270 carers in this county.

An earlier interview based study on carers in East Sussex undertaken by the Tavistock Institute (Carer Stress and Carer Support, 1988) had indicated that carers benefit from a 'package of care'. Such a 'package' might include support from a number of sources – statutory, voluntary, informal or privately paid for. This study aims to provide statistical data on the nature of support received by carers from eleven DHSS funded schemes in East Sussex and feedback on the schemes established under the Demonstration District Initiative.

2 Methods

The research was conducted by way of a questionnaire designed to be relatively simple and quick to complete. The questionnaires were given to 295 carers who were receiving support from one of eleven of the Demonstration District's funded schemes, selected on the basis of variety of service offered and geographical range in terms of the urban and rural dimension of East Sussex.

The questionnaire comprised four main sections. The first on demographic and lifestyle characteristics, based loosely on the questions from the 1985 General Household Survey. The second on possible problems experienced by carers. The third on the nature of community support and the fourth on the help received from the relevant funded scheme.

The questionnaire was returned by 170 carers, 57.6% of the 295 sent out. It was analysed by computer using a statistical programme for social scientists. This work was undertaken at Brighton Polytechnic with the kind assistance of Peter Frost, Roman Foley and David Leach.

3 Demographic characteristics of the carer and their dependants

1 The Carers

In this sample of 170 carers, 166 were looking after one person whilst three carers were looking after two and one was caring for three people.

Over two-thirds were women, some 70% of the sample.

This figure is consistent with a number of other studies and with the Equal Opportunities Commission 1982 estimate that, in the nation as a whole, there are three times as many women carers as men. It is, however, a far higher ratio than that described in the General Household Survey – possibly attributable to the characteristics of this sample. Most of the voluntary services involved were catered for carers looking after people with considerable levels of disability; even within the general household survey, the numbers of women looking after very disabled dependants were higher than men.

A large number of the carers were in older age groups reflecting the high proportion of this group in the country. Whilst a large number, 33% were in the 45–64 year old bracket, 51% were aged over 65 and almost a quarter, 23% were aged over 75 years. Over a fifth, 21.2% were carers aged 75 years and over looking after a dependant of 75 years or over.

The largest group (49.4%) were people looking after their spouse followed by those looking after children. (22.1%)

As might be expected, the proportion of carers looking after a spouse increased with age. Table 1.2 shows the percentages of carers in five age bands who were looking after a dependant in the relationship categories above.

Table 1. *Percentage of carers looking after family members, relatives and friends or neighbours by age*

Age of Carer	Relationship to dependant				
	spouse	child(ren)	parent(s) or parent(s)-in-law	other relative	friend(s) neigh-bour(s)
20–29 years	—	100.0%	—	—	—
30–44 years	4.3%	87.0%	4.3%	4.3%	—
45–64 years	29.8%	24.6%	36.8%	3.5%	3.5%
65–74 years	76.6%	4.3%	10.6%	2.1%	4.3%
75 years & over	77.5%	2.5%	2.5%	12.5%	5.0%
Total percentage of sample	50%	22.1%	16.9%	5.2%	3.5%

2 *The Dependants*

As Table 3.1 shows, almost one half of carers had dependants aged 75 years and over. The ratio of the sexes was roughly equal.

Table 2.1 *(a) sex and (b) age of dependant*

(a) sex of dependant	%
male	47.1
female	50.0
non specified	2.9
(b) age of dependant	**%**
0 to 4	2.9
5 to 15	11.6
16 to 44	7.6
45 to 64	13.4
65 to 74	18.0
75 or over	44.8

It was rare for a man to be caring for anyone other than his wife as shown in Table 2.2. However, some five male carers were looking after a parent or parent-in-law and four were caring for a friend or neighbour.

Table 2.2 *Sex of Carer by relationship to dependant*

relationship to dependant	sex of carer	
	male	female
spouse	19.4%	30.0%
child	0.6%	21.2%
parent or parent-in-law	2.9%	12.4%
other relative	.6%	4.7%
friend or neighbour	2.4%	1.2%
non-specified	.6%	.6%
total percentage by sex of carer	26.5%	70.0%

The questionnaire sought to distinguish between those who had a physical disability and those with mental or psychological problems as this would affect the type of care required. Given the nature of this sample with a high proportion of dependants aged over 75 years it was not always easy for carers completing the questionnaire to distinguish a specific illness or disability other than general 'old age'. In categorising the responses to this question, mental illness and mental handicap were grouped together in terms of 'mental disability' although it was recognised that they have different needs. This was in accordance with the General Household Survey where, as noted, many carers were ''unable to make the distinction''.

Just over a third of carers (37.8%) were looking after someone with a physical disability only, and almost a quarter were both physically and mentally disabled or ill in some way (Table 2.3). This was by contrast with the General Household Survey in which 73% had only physical disabilities. This probably reflects the nature of the schemes through which the carers were contacted: at one end there were two schemes for mentally handicapped children and at the other there were several schemes caring mainly for the elderly, with one specifically for those suffering from Alzheimer's Disease.

Table 2.3 *Disability of dependant*

physical disability	37.8%
mental disability	20.3%
physical and mental disability	23.8%
old age	12.8%
other	1.7%

4 The nature of care

This section explores the time devoted to caring by carers, the type of help they are providing and the level of dependency of those they are looking after.

Number of years caring

Some 57.5% had been caring for their dependant for over five years including 26.7% of over ten years. This figure was higher than that estimated in the General Household Survey where 43% had been looking after their dependant for over five years.

Table 3.1 *Number of years caring for dependant*

number of years	%
under 1 year	4.7
1–2 years	12.2
3–5 years	23.3
5–10 years	30.8
10 years or over	26.7

Time spent on caring activities

Carers were asked to indicate the time spent on average looking after their dependant each week. As Table 3.2 indicates, 89% of carers devoted at least 50 hours per week to caring and only 2.3% less than 20 hours. This contrasts with the General Household Survey where the equivalent figures were 14% and 37%; reflecting very clearly the more dependent nature of the people looked after by carers using the schemes in this survey. On the basis of the original General Household Survey estimate, it may be concluded that there are upwards of 10,958 carers in East Sussex devoting at least 50 hours per week to looking after their relative or friend.

Table 3.2. *Number of hours caring per week*

number of hours	%
over 50	89.0
20-49	7.0
under 20	2.3

Types of help

Almost all the carers (94.7%) helped their dependant with personal care activities such as dressing, bathing, washing.

Table 3.3 *Types of help given to dependant(s)*

type of help	%
personal help (e.g. washing, using the toilet)	94.7
help with paperwork and financial matters	80.6

Table 3.3 *Types of help given to dependant(s)* (Cont'd)

other practical help (shopping, preparing meals, etc.)	97.6
keeping them company	95.3
taking out: for walk, to see friends, etc.	76.5
giving medicines	87.6
keeping an eye on dependant	94.7

The level of dependency of the people the carers were looking after in this sample was further demonstrated in the questionnaire as to whether the dependant could be left alone should the carer wish to go out for a couple of hours. Over three-quarters of carers (77.6%) responded that their dependant could not be left without someone looking after them. When asked how difficult it would be to arrange for someone else to look after their dependant for a couple of hours, 28.8% indicated that it would be very difficult, 40% quite difficult; 20% hadn't tried.

Taken as a whole the quantitative information derived from the first section of the questionnaire reveals that the carers in this sample are looking after people with a very high level of dependency and need. The majority had been doing so for many years. Over a half were aged over 65 years and could themselves be suffering from failing health.

What happens to such carers? What are the emotional and physical implications for them? How far are they being supported by the statutory agencies? What sort of support can they derive from alternative schemes in the voluntary sector? These questions are explored in the following three sections of the report.

5 Problems experienced by carers

A list of possible problems was drawn up based upon difficulties reported by carers in the interview focused Tavistock Institute research on Carer Stress and Carer Support. Carers were asked to indicate those which were a problem to them and to what degree (constant, sometimes or hardly ever). The problems could loosely be categorised into four types: emotional, physical or concerned with a sense of isolation or not knowing where to get help or information. The levels of difficulty and stress are detailed in Table 4.1.

Many carers reported experiencing constant problems across the board.

Areas of particular difficulty, indicated as a 'constant problem' by some 40% of carers' were tiredness, stress and nerves, having time for themselves, being able to get out to do shopping or visit friends and worry about the future. One of the most important factors affecting the carers' ability to cope and, indeed, to carry on caring, is their own state of health, often closely linked to their emotional state and affected by the level of stress they are under. Almost a third of carers (31.2%) in this study reported that their own health was a 'constant problem' and a further 44% that their health was 'sometimes' a problem.

A further factor in levels of emotional stress may be the extent of contact and support from family and friends. A number of carers indicated difficulties in keeping in touch with family and friends (18.8% a 'constant problem' and 29.4% 'sometimes' a problem). Strain in relationships with other family members was also revealed, with some 15.3% indicating this to be a 'constant problem' and 24.7% reporting this to be 'sometimes a problem'.

Closely related to the carers' state of health is their ability to cope with the physical demands of caring. Approximately 30% of the carers in this sample indicated that they experienced 'constant problems' in coping with the physical tasks of bathing, toileting and lifting or carrying their dependants. The strain of dealing with heavy physical demands affects the carer's health and associated strength and increases the problem. Many carers are, of course, elderly themselves.

Table 4.1 *Problems experienced by carers by severity of problem*

Type of problem	constant problem %	sometimes a problem %	hardly ever a problem %	No response/ not relevant %
• House cleaning, house & garden maintenance	30.6	34.7	14.7	20.0
• Lifting or carrying the dependant	27.1	35.9	15.9	21.2
• Bathing the dependant	32.9	24.7	19.6	22.9
• Toileting the dependant	29.4	25.3	23.5	21.8
• The house (e.g. stairs unmanageable)	11.8	15.3	33.3	39.4
• Not enough space in the house	8.2	14.7	44.1	32.9

Table 4.1 *Problems experienced by carers by severity of problem* (Cont'd)

Type of problem	constant problem %	sometimes a problem %	hardly ever a problem %	No response/ not relevant %
• Own health e.g. back problem	31.2	44.1	9.4	15.3
• Getting out for shopping/ visits	39.4	41.2	7.6	11.8
• Personal time for care	41.8	38.2	6.5	13.5
• Keeping in touch with family or friends	18.8	29.4	27.1	24.7
• Strain between other family members	15.3	24.7	31.6	28.2
• Worry about future	47.6	25.3	12.4	14.7
• Lack of sleep at night	27.1	48.8	9.4	14.7
• Constant tiredness, stress, nerves	39.4	41.2	8.2	11.2
• Difficult behaviour of dependant	24.7	38.2	23.5	13.5
• No one to talk things over with	16.5	26.5	32.9	21.1
• Not enough money to cover bills and basic needs	9.4	18.2	42.9	29.4
• Not knowing where to get help	6.5	24.7	34.1	34.7
• Doubts about carrying on caring	15.9	30.0	23.5	30.6

In the Tavistock Institute study on 'Carer Stress and Carer Support' almost all the carers interviewed wanted to continue caring for as long as they were physically capable. In the present study a number of carers indicated that they had doubts as to whether they were able to do so. 15.9% reported that doubts about carrying on caring was a constant problem and a further 30% that this was sometimes a problem. As was mentioned earlier, the carers in this sample are clearly experiencing a high level of both emotional and physical stress. Critical questions arise as to how far they are being currently supported and can their situations be significantly improved?

6 The carers' views of community support

Despite such stresses, the carers in the sample were carrying on, but a major factor affecting their ability to do so is the availability of both practical and social/emotional support.

The third section of the questionnaire was designed to examine the levels of support carers were receiving from the statutory services, from voluntary groups and from family and friends. A list of possible sources of support was drawn up and carers were asked to indicate those from which they had received some help and to rate how helpful that had been (i.e. very helpful, quite helpful or not very helpful).

The carers in this sample were probably receiving more support than many other carers, in so far as they were selected because they were using a voluntary carer service funded under the DHSS initiative. The voluntary schemes may also have advised carers of the range of formal services, including social security benefits, available to them. Similarly, the spread of information about the funded voluntary schemes may well have encouraged the statutory agencies to refer known carers to wider sources of support.

Table 5.1 shows that the carers in this sample were receiving support from a variety of formal and informal sources. The data is, of course, open to interpretation. For example, it may be argued that the fact that 63.5% are receiving or have received help from a district or community nurse shows that a high level of support is being offered by this service. But was this support sufficient in terms of time and relief given?

Table 5.1 *Sources of support and degree of helpfulness*

	Service not received/ not relevant %	Carers using service found it		
		not very helpful %	quite helpful %	very helpful %
Aids & minor adaptations	34.1	9.8	22.3	67.9
Major adaptations	72.9	10.8	34.8	54.4
Home help	73.5	20	20	60
Meals on wheels	87.6	42.8	9.6	47.6
District/community nurse	36.5	11.2	26.8	62

Table 5.1 *Sources of support and degree of helpfulness* (Cont'd)

	Service not received/ not relevant %	Carers using service found it		
		not very helpful %	quite helpful %	very helpful %
O.T.	70.6	22	38	40
Laundry service	91.8	35.3	22	42.7
Physiotherapist	69.4	24.8	36.6	38.6
Relief care service	42.9	6.4	26.7	66.9
Respite care	60.6	19.4	22.4	58.2
Day centre	57.6	13.9	19.6	66.5
School/adult training centre	82.9	10.5	14	75.5
Social worker/welfare officer	55.9	18.4	26.7	54.7
G.P.	20.0	12.5	29.4	58.1
Hospital consultant	51.8	18.2	39	42.8
C.P.N.	92.4	38.1	15.8	46.1
Carer support group	35.9	3.7	18.3	78
Counsellor or psychologist	90.0	65	23	12
Financial support	14.1	1.3	18.5	80.2
Voluntary orgs	55.9	4	14.7	81.3
Friends/neighbours	40.6	12.6	45.7	41.7
Family	57.1	9.5	31.5	59

6.1 The Health Service

The general practitioner and district/community nurse were the most frequently cited sources of support from the 'professional' services. Both were rated fairly highly in terms of their degree of helpfulness. Some 58.1% of carers rated their GP as being 'very helpful' and 62% the district nurse in similar terms. Just under a half indicated that they had received help from a hospital consultant (48%) but only 42.8% of these rated this as very helpful. Approximately 30% of carers had received help (for their dependants) from a physiotherapist with only 38.6% rating this service as 'very helpful'. Still lower, only 7% had received help from a community psychiatric nurse (CPN) with only 46% describing this as 'very helpful'. This latter figure seems low given that 44% of the dependants in this study were suffering from a mental disability or from both a physical and mental disability.

6.2 *The Social Services*

Some 43% of carers indicated that their dependant was attending or had had contact with a day centre, and a further 17% with a school or adult training centre. 66.5% rated the day centre as being very helpful and 75.5% the school or adult training centre. Such services can provide the carers with time to themselves or time to undertake tasks they may be unable to do when their dependant is with them.

Practical help in the form of special aids and adaptations is a service which may provide invaluable help to a carer looking after a disabled or frail dependant. 66% of carers had received some help in the form of aids and minor adaptations, with 67.9% rating this as very helpful. 27% had had major adaptations to their home undertaken with 54.4% rating this as very helpful. Less than a third of the sample indicated that they had received help from an occupational therapist: this may be attributable to misunderstanding about the term.

The Home Help service has traditionally focused on people living alone. 27% of carers in this sample indicated that they had received help from this service, although this figure includes private home helps, mentioned by a few carers. The service was found to be very helpful by 60% of those receiving the service. A fairly small number of carers received meals on wheels for their dependants or, indeed, themselves. Only 47.6% of these rated this service as very helpful.

Carers were also asked to indicate whether they had received any help from a social worker or welfare officer. 44% indicated that they had had contact, with 54.7% rating this as very helpful. However, carers did not always distinguish between help that came from statutory or voluntary services, so it is possible that the organisers of the funded carer support schemes may well have been regarded as welfare officers. It is interesting to note that counsellors and psychologists were rarely found to be either very helpful (12%) or helpful (23%), although these were used by so few carers that these figures cannot be seen as very reliable.

Respite care in the form of short-stays in residential homes or via the Family Link Scheme for mentally handicapped children is a growing resource in East Sussex. Some 40% of carers indicated that they had received help from this type of service, with 58.2% rating this as being very helpful. This statistic also includes respite care offered in hospitals.

6.3 *Voluntary Services*

The services included in the questionnaire under this category were: help from a voluntary organisation, carer support group and sitting or relief care service. It was a somewhat loose category since the statutory services also run carer support groups and relief care services. All carers in this sample were receiving help from a voluntary organisation in the form of one or more of the funded schemes. However, only 45% gave any such indication which may be due to a misunderstanding of the terms or lack of realisation that the schemes were run by voluntary organisations. Some 64% indicated that they had received help from a carer support group with 78% rating this as very helpful. 57% had received help from a sitting or relief care service, with 66.9% indicating this as very helpful.

6.4 *Informal Support*

Carers were also asked whether they received support from family, friends and neighbours and to rate how helpful that support was felt to be.

Some 60% indicated that they were helped by friends and neighbours. 45% of these found this to be very helpful and a similar number (41.7%), quite helpful. Support from family was, perhaps surprisingly, less common. Some 57% of carers gave no indication of support from their own family although 59% of those who did have support, rated this as being very helpful. A number of interpretations could be placed on this including higher expectations placed on one's family and the fact that many carers indicated that relatives, including sons and daughters, simply lived too far away. Others indicated that their relatives could not believe or accept the deterioration in the person the carer was looking after.

6.5 *Financial Support*

This refers to support form DHSS benefits, including attendance allowance, invalid care allowance and mobility allowance. In this sample 86% of carers indicated that they were receiving help in the form of benefits and 80% rated this as being very helpful. It may well be that through contact with the organisers of the funded schemes the carers in this sample were alerted to their possible entitlements. A relatively small proportion (9.4%) of carers indicated in the previous section of the questionnaire that having too little money to cover bills and basic needs was a constant problem.

7 The carers' views of the funded schemes

The final section of the questionnaire explores the kind of needs met by the voluntary schemes funded under the Department of Health initiative and how helpful carers perceived the services to be. The services funded under this initiative are listed in Appendix 1, with stars against those which sent questionnaires to their carers.

Ten different ways in which services might have been found helpful were listed and carers were asked to indicate whether these applied to the service they received (i.e. very helpful, quite helpful, doesn't apply). Carers were also asked to indicate what they had particularly liked and not liked about the service or had found made it difficult to use.

Most of the schemes focused on one service but a number offered two or more. Carers often reported being helped on a number of different dimensions, even when the main aim of the service was one specific kind of support. However, part of the strength of individual services were that they met specific needs that enabled them to complement other services provided elsewhere. As was noted in the Tavistock Institute Paper on 'Carer Stress and Carer Support': ''the evaluation of any one service must also take into account the fact that it may be the total 'package' of care that makes the difference to the carer, not any one particular item within the package. A sitting service without the information service that referred the carer or the support group that enabled the carer to cope with the guilt engendered by using the service may have made little difference'' (Susan Hodgson and Dione Hills).

7.1 Age Concern Saturday Club

This scheme is a social club for carers and their dependants where both can meet others with broadly similar problems in a relaxed, informal atmosphere. A paid organiser is assisted by voluntary helpers.

Carers using this scheme who returned the questionnaire (63%) found the service to be very helpful in a range of ways, most frequently appreciating the social aspects. 'Someone to talk to', 'helped in feeling less stressed and anxious' and 'helped in meeting others with similar problems'. Help in receiving information about other services, benefits, etc. was also indicated by a number of carers. Carers particularly liked the friendly, helpful concern, the companionship and the understanding offered and the fact that both carer and dependant could use the service together.

7.2 *Alzheimer's Disease Society Sitting Service*

This scheme provides paid sitters to enable carers of people suffering from Alzheimer's Disease to have a break. The 14 carers (35%) who returned the questionnaire, again most frequently described the service as very helpful, not only in giving them a break but also relieving their loneliness and isolation; 'having personal time, time to do other things', having someone to talk to', 'helped in feeling less stressed and anxious'. General comments included the helpfulness, kindliness and friendliness of the staff. The only criticisms were from 2 carers who wished that the service was more available, especially at short notice and in the evenings.

7.3 *Carousel*

This scheme offered a weekly after school club for children with mental handicaps, thereby enabling parents (carers) to have additional time for themselves. The scheme also offered carers a massage, movement and relaxation group and enabled carers to make a video to present their experiences to others. Although half of the carers returning the questionnaire indicated that the scheme had been very helpful in 'having personal time, time to do other things', 'giving reliable care to their dependant' and 'helped in feeling less stressed and anxious', demand for the service was not very high and the grant for the after school club was not renewed.

7.4 *Battle Carers' Centre*

This scheme offers respite to carers through a day care provision for their dependant and more recently (since July 1988) a sitting service. The scheme has also set up a carers' support group and the day centre offers general support and information to carers with a member of staff specialising in this. The day centre is sited in part of rural East Sussex where no other such provision exists.

The thirteen carers (65%) who returned the questionnaire indicated that they had found the scheme gave 'reliable care to their relative/friend', 'gave their relative/friend an interest/someone to talk to' and 'made coping a bit easier'. Carers also indicated that they had found the service helpful in enabling them to have 'someone to talk to', 'giving information about other services, benefits, etc.' and in feeling 'less stressed and anxious'. Carers particularly commented upon the friendliness, kindliness and concern of the staff. The only criticism was of transport difficulties.

7.5 *Crossroads Schemes*

These schemes provide paid and trained care attendants to look after the disabled person in order to give their carer a break. The 41 carers who returned the questionnaire indicated that they had found the service to be very helpful in giving 'reliable care to their relative/friend' followed by 'making coping a bit easier', 'helping to feel less stressed and anxious', 'having personal time, time to do other things', 'having someone to talk to' and 'giving their relative/friend an interest, someone to talk to'. Carers also commented on the efficiency, reliability and friendliness of the care attendants and the scheme organiser. Comment was also made on the care taken in matching help to need. Three carers made criticisms, one hoping for more care attendant time, another that her child's needs were too complex for the care attendant to provide more than 'light relief' and the third wanting someone to take out her multiply disabled son rather than just coming in and sitting with him.

7.6 *Eastbourne Parents Action Group*

This scheme offers a 'babysitting' service to parents (carers) of young, mentally handicapped children. Regular meetings are also held enabling parents to meet others in a similar situation. The questionnaire was returned by 17 carers (85%). The social aspect was most frequently commented upon: approximately a half indicated that they had found the service to be very helpful in 'meeting other with similar problems', 'having someone to talk to', 'making coping a bit easier'. Similar numbers found the scheme gave 'reliable care to their relative/friend'. A smaller proportion indicated that they had found the service very helpful in 'giving personal time/time to do other things; and 'helping to feel less stressed and anxious'. Carers also commented on the reliability of the care offered and the benefits of no 'red tape'. One carer commented that because she was unable to attend meetings she had nobody to talk over problems with. Another felt that the particular problem of her child were not understood and another that the participants of the meetings tended to ''clan''.

7.7 *The Association of Carers, Hastings and St Leonards*

This scheme operates a sitting service with volunteer sitters and paid organisers. The questionnaire was returned by 11 carers (52%). Just over a half found the service to be very helpful in 'giving personal time, time to do other things', followed by 'giving reliable care to their relative/friend' and making 'coping a bit easier'. Carers also commented on the reliability of the service and the kindly and friendly manner of the scheme organisers.

Two carers made criticisms, one that the service was not available at short notice and the other that his sitter would not make hot drinks.

7.8 *Hove Carers' Centre*

This scheme offers advice and information to carers at the centre and over the telephone, a telephone 'helpline' and also provides coffee mornings to enable carers to meet one another and to talk over shared problems. It is also a proactive scheme in highlighting the needs of carers to the wider community, including local statutory agencies. The emotional support provided by the service was on the whole seen as being of primary importance. Of the 16 carers (53%) who returned the questionnaire, a large proportion indicated that they found having someone to talk to 'very helpful'. This was followed by help in 'meeting others with similar problems', help in 'feeling less stressed and anxious' and help in making 'coping a bit easier'. Just over a third indicated that they found the service to be very helpful in providing information about other services or their relative/friends' illness and how to manage this. Carers made particular note of the friendly and caring approach of the staff. The only criticism related to the siting of the office – on the first floor of a building up steep stairs.

7.9 *Lewes Area Relief Care Scheme*

This scheme offers a relief care service using paid and trained staff on both an emergency and routine basis. 14 carers (88%) using this service returned the questionnaire. Of these, a high proportion indicated that they found the provision of 'reliable care to their relative or friend' to be very helpful. Also highly rated were help in giving the carer personal time, time to do other things and 'giving their relative or friend someone to talk to'. Over a half indicated that the service was very helpful in helping to 'make coping a bit easier', with a slightly lower number responding that the service was very helpful in providing information about other service, benefits, etc. As with many of the other schemes, carers particularly noted the friendliness, reliability and helpfulness of the staff. One carer commented that the staff were always at the end of the telephone if needed and noted that they were always willing to listen to problems and offer advice. This same carer was the only one to make any criticism – that the 'care attendant' that his parents had been used to had to give up the work, and they found it hard to adapt to a new person.

7.10 *Polegate and District Carers' Scheme*

This scheme offers a relief sitting service, counselling and support, information about benefits and local services and also a number of carers' support groups across the area. The relief sitting service is provided by voluntary helpers and paid sessional workers. 29 carers (86%) returned the questionnaire. The sources of help reported as most helpful were, firstly 'information about other services, benefits, etc'., followed by 'reduction of stress and anxiety, having someone to talk to', 'making coping a bit easier' and 'meeting others in a similar situation'. Just over a third of carers indicated that they found the service very helpful in providing reliable care to their relative/friend, providing information on their relative/friend's illness/handicap and how to manage this. As described above, this scheme is a broadly ranging one. As for the other schemes, favourable comments were made about the friendliness, sympathy and willingness of the staff to offer help and the reliability of that help. The only indirect criticism was that the sitting service should offer more hours.

9 Conclusion

This study presents a broad range of data on a sample of carers who could be described in terms of being at the sharp end of caring. They are looking after people with an extremely high level of dependency. Many are experiencing great difficulties in carrying out the various caring tasks and are experiencing high levels of stress. This is so despite receiving support from a range of statutory, informal, privately paid for or voluntary services.

For many, such support can make a vital contribution towards making their situation more manageable and enabling them to cope. It would seem that these carer focussed schemes are meeting a number of important needs; needs that may not be met elsewhere. Nevertheless, there are limitations. As was pointed out by a number of the carers, more help of this nature is needed, with greater time flexibility to include a night service when required. More resources are needed to fund such an extension and to develop further similar schemes.

Many indicated that the support received had been very helpful in reducing stress and anxiety, allowing personal time, making coping a bit easier and, significantly, in giving them someone to talk to. Caring can be a lonely and extremely isolating occupation. Having someone to talk to may well be a factor in reducing levels of stress and anxiety and the carers' ability to cope.

A large proportion also commented upon the reliability and efficiency of their service. This is of vital importance for a carer entrusting their dependant to the care of another. Many carers commented that the service had given their dependant an interest or someone to talk to. This is also important in reducing guilt and allowing the carer to feel that their dependant's needs are also being met. Indeed, a number of carers commented that their dependant found difficulty in dealing with new people and that they had been able to use the service because it was acceptable to their dependant.

A large majority of carers who completed the questionnaire made only positive comments about the services they received. As was pointed out in the earlier Tavistock Institute paper on 'Carer Stress and Carer Support', carers' expectations of help tend to be low. Possible explanations of this are that they have assumed they must cope on their own or that they experienced earlier on that help was simply not available. In terms of criticising services, carers may be anxious that if they do so then that source of help might be withdrawn. The most frequent criticism made by carers was that they would have liked more of the help offered by their individual services, more hours, more days, more availability at short notice and an extension of the service to cover nights in the case of sitting and care attendant schemes. More resources are needed to enable such schemes to provide a broader, more flexible service.

Finally, as was referred to earlier, there are upwards of 10,958 people in this county devoting at least 50 hours per week to caring. The carers who have received support via the DHSS initiative in East Sussex are only the tip of the iceberg. There remains a large unmet need.

In terms of the help provided by the eleven DHSS funded voluntary schemes described, it is clear that carers certainly appreciate such support. Being able to leave the person they are looking after for a few hours or simply having someone sympathetic to talk to may ease the burden considerably.

Such voluntary schemes should be seen as an essential part of the range of services for carers, the total 'package of care', and should be carefully co-ordinated with them. In relation to the planning of services, proper and real recognition needs to be given to the voluntary sector in providing such support. A number of lessons may be learned.

Appendix B1

Services funded by Caring for the Carers, East Sussex

Purpose of Grant	Size of annual grant	Non cash Subsidies	Staffing	Level of service to carers
Open meetings,	£200–£500	Charity rates for hire of premises	Staff from other agencies involved	Between 50 and 100 carers and professionals involved
Summer Play schemes (2)	£870–3000	Use of school premises, transport,	Temporary play scheme staff	Two weeks day-time respite for parents of handicapped children
Carer group	£500			Grant to cover admin and outings
Carers' Co-op drop in centre run by carers of people with: mental health problems for information and support	£1,600	Health Auth. premises and support from NSF	Volunteers	Approx. 5 visits a week from carers
***Eastbourne Parents Action Group,** babysitting for 0–5 year old physically handicapped children	£6000	SSD support and advice, service run from parent's home	3 paid baby sitters	13 carers use service regularly
***Age Concern Saturday Club**	£6500	SSD premises, AC supervision and office premises, Red Cross & SSD transport	Part time organiser + volunteers	12 carers and dependants use club each Saturday
***Carousel After School Club** for children with disabilities	£10,000	Carousel premises, payroll and support	2 part-time creative therapists	After school respite care, support to parents

Services funded by Caring for the Carers, East Sussex (Cont'd)

Purpose of Grant	Size of annual grant	Non cash Subsidies	Staffing	Level of service to carers
Wealdon MENCAP Family Support worker-information parents workshops, helps parents buy in relief care	£15000	MENCAP supervision and payroll, SSD Accom.	Full time family support worker	Support etc. to 20 families
***Lewes Area Relief Care Scheme** mainly for elderly people	£15000	LA payroll, staff work for home	Part time coordinator + 4 paid helpers	20 carers receive 10–12 hours a month
***Polegate and District Carer Scheme** worker gives support, information, development of carer groups and sitting services for carers of elderly physically handicapped people	£18000	SSD accom. & payroll, support and training of care staff	Full time development worker + 4 paid sitters +4 volunteers	10 carers receive 3 hours relief a week, plus others receiving personal and group support
***Alzheimer's Disease Society** relief care scheme and information and support	£21000	ADS payroll and supervision	Full time organiser + part time relief carers	28 carers use scheme each week
***Association of Carers** Sitting service using volunteers	£18000	SSD premises	2 part time organisers + 22 volunteer sitters	21 carers receive 3 hrs relief care each week
***Crossroads Care Attendant Schemes** (3 – one in each health district) practical help and respite for wide range of carers	£25000–£50000	LA and HA accom. National Crossroads training and support	Part time coordinators + care attendants	10–15 hours help per month per carer
***Hove Carers' Centre** Information and support through drop in centre, mobile desk, help line and development work	£48000	CVS supervision and payroll	2 full time 2 part time staff	20 carers drop in to centre
***Battle Carers' Centre** day care, sitting service, support group, general information and support	£32000	SSD back-up (OT and social work, transport) HA premises	Full time organiser + 3 part time care attendants	20 carers use centre each week

Appendix C

SUPPORTING CARERS IN SANDWELL
Report of a survey of carers using services funded by Sandwell Caring for Carers Project

Roger Page

CONTENTS

Introduction

In the last five years, the role of informal carers has come to the forefront of attention because of a growing crisis in society caused by an increase in the number of people giving and needing care in the home. This has been partly because of demographic factors: the increase in numbers of elderly, and the decrease in the numbers in a position to provide this care. However, there have also been political and economic factors: a decrease in the number of places in institutional care, and a policy move towards maintaining people in their own homes or other community based provision.

In 1986 the Department of Health (under the then Secretary of State Norman Fowler) set up the 'Demonstration Districts for Informal Carers' programme to investigate one dimension of community care; the capacity of the voluntary sector to provide support to informal carers. Sandwell Caring for Carers was one of three consortia of voluntary and statutory representatives set up to distribute grants to voluntary organisations. The consortium used its budget of £600,000 to fund 8 carer services, a brief description of which is given in Table 1. This consortium was particularly concerned to see that the views, concerns and experiences of the carers who were using the services that were grant aided should not be lost. It decided to carry out an 'opinion poll of carer views' using a carer support profile drawn up in collaboration with the Tavistock Institute researchers who were monitoring the whole programme. The profile was distributed to carers via the 8 services, but the completed questionnaires were returned to the consortium itself, via a stamped addressed envelope, to ensure that carers would not feel inhibited from making criticism by the thought that staff in the services would see their reply.

The overall response rate was 45%, but the different numbers of users of different services meant that many more questionnaires were returned for some services than others (see Table 2). There was also a different response rate for different services, in particular, those dealing with quite elderly users had rather lower rates, which suggests that the picture of this group is less representative than some of the other groups. Some caution should therefore be used in the the interpretation of the tables.

The profile covered four dimensions.

1 demographic profile,

2 carers' difficulties,

3 their use of statutory and voluntary services, and

4 their attitude to grant aided services that they were receiving.

The questionnaire was analysed with the help of Sandwell College of Further Education.

Analysis of results

1 Demographic Profile of Carers

The first part of the carer profile included several questions taken from the General Household Survey of carers carried out in 1985. These were included in order to see how far the carers using schemes were similar or different to a national sample of carers. Table 3 shows the general profile of carers receiving help from Sandwell services was not dissimilar, in terms of age and sex, from the carers found by the General Household Survey who were caring for over 20 hours a week. However, because three out of the eight services surveyed were providing services for handicapped young people, there was a higher proportion of carers in the Sandwell survey who were in the age range 30–44, and who were looking after children.

On the whole, carers receiving the carer services in Sandwell were looking after people with a higher level of dependency than the carers in the national sample who were looking after someone in their own home, or caring for over 20 hours a week. A higher proportion using Sandwell services were spending over 50 hours a week looking after their dependant, fewer could leave their dependants for a short time without finding someone else to look after them, and a larger proportion had difficulty finding sitters to replace themselves if they did want to go out. More were required to carry out a whole range of care tasks, from help with personal care, giving medicine, keeping an eye on their dependant (to make sure they didn't come to any harm) and help with practical tasks. A higher proportion (40%) had been caring for over ten years. Proportionately more had dependants who were suffering from mental disabilities (with or without physical disabilities as well) or who were suffering from general frailty and disability connected with old age.

Table 3A gives a break down on some variables by scheme. This shows that the carers receiving help from schemes fell into three main groups: those using services for young handicapped people (Sandcastle, ICAN and Sandwell Multi-Handicap Group), those receiving services that were mainly for the elderly (Hately Heath, Age Concern, Akrill), and those receiving services that cater for all age groups (Crossroads and CARES).

Carers receiving services from schemes for younger disabled people were mainly looking after sons or daughters who were under 16; they themselves were mostly between 20 and 44 years old. Most were unable to leave their dependants without someone else looking after them, but unlike carers of older people, many did not find it too difficult to find a sitter to replace them if they went out. A high proportion of the children that they were looking after were suffering from mental handicaps, with or without physical handicaps as well.

Most of the carers completing the questionnaires from these schemes were women, probably because mothers are usually designated as the main carer of younger children. Carers using ICAN had the most difficulty in finding alternative care for their handicapped youngster. This was a service for Asian families, and this may have reflected differing cultural attitudes towards handicap and parental responsibilities; alternatively, it may have indicated that this group had particular difficulty in gaining access to any available services. Sandwell Multi Handicap Group had more carers of adult handicapped sons and daughters using their services. Crossroads and Akrill Day Centre both cater for non elderly ill and disabled people as well as the elderly, but both, like Age Concern, were used by a high proportion of elderly carers looking after elderly and very elderly dependants. Mostly these were carers looking after spouses or parents. The dependants using Akrill appeared to be the most able of those using these three services: hardly any were suffering from mental disorders, nearly two thirds could be left without a sitter, and fewer needed help with personal care. This probably reflects the nature of the care provided: dependants need to be relatively able to use a day centre, although the centre can cater for people with relatively severe physical and mental difficulties, and provides help with practical caring tasks such as bathing and chiropody.

Carers using Crossroads and C.A.R.E.S. were most likely to still be in part time or full time work, and were mostly caring for dependants with physical rather than mental handicaps. Overall, although C.A.R.E.S. caters for a wide cross section of carers, the level of dependency of the people they are looking after does not appear to be much less than that of carers using sitting or respite care schemes. A high proportion, two thirds, were caring for over 50 hours per week, and similar numbers were unable to leave their dependant without a sitter. However, a much higher proportion of these carers were not living in the same house as their dependant and some were living further away than the immediate neighbourhood, and some had dependants in residential homes or hostels. This reflects the fact that this was a general information and enquiry service: some enquirers may have been considering taking on a greater level of care: for example, their dependant moving into the carers' home.

2. Problems experienced by carers

Table 4 shows the kind of problems experienced by carers. Difficulties with managing the physical side of caring: laundry, house cleaning, and lifting, bathing and toileting their dependants were particularly a problem with carers using the Age Concern service, mainly because of the age of these carers and their dependants, but also a problem for carers of the younger physically and mentally handicapped. Over a third of carers using all services had health problems of their own, but particularly carers using C.A.R.E.S., Crossroads and Barnardos, where nearly half had health problems. Having time to themselves, getting out of the house, and keeping in touch with other members of the family and friends (generally factors that lead to isolation amongst carers) affected over half the carers, and was particularly severe amongst carers using Age Concern, Crossroads, Sandcastle and ICAN.

Stress factors: lack of sleep, strain amongst other family members, constant tiredness and worry about the future were a constant problem for about a third of carers, particularly carers using C.A.R.E.S., Crossroads and Sandcastle. Lack of information about services, lack of money, and lack of anyone to talk to about the problems of caring was a severe problem for about 20% of carers, particularly for carers using Akrill, C.A.R.E.S. and ICAN. Half the carers using Barnardos had money difficulties.

3. Receipt of other services

Table 5 shows that quite a high proportion of the carers using the grant aided services were not in receipt of any other services such as adaptations of their house, home helps, meals on wheels, or occupational therapists. The only services or help received by over 50% were from minor aids (walkers etc), Social Security benefits and G.P.s. Nurses, social workers and hospital consultants were helping just under half of the carers. A few mentioned voluntary services and sitting services; these were probably the grant aided schemes. Just under half went to a carer support group, but these were mainly run in conjunction with the Caring for Carer schemes.

In terms of satisfaction, or feeling helped by services (Table 5A) voluntary services came out very well, with around 75% liking their sitting services or carer group, and no one expressing dissatisfaction with voluntary services.

Benefits were felt to be very helpful by most people in receipt of these, and respite and day care services were felt to be helpful by around 66% of those who received any support from these. Schools were found very helpful by most of the 89 carers who had handicapped children of school age.

Services that were found to be less helpful were meals on wheels, occupational therapists, laundry services, community psychiatric nurses and counsellors and psychologists. Since these were all services that are in quite limited supply, it is likely that the limited quantity of these services, rather than the quality, was the source of frustration. Given some of the assumptions that are made about the kind of help that friends and family can provide, it is worth recording that over a third apparently received no help from this source, and where help was received, it was recorded by a relatively low proportion (40% and 49% respectively) as very helpful. However, it is possible that expectations of family and friends were higher than expectations of formal services.

4. *Satisfaction with Carer services*

Most of the carers receiving the services provided by schemes grant aided by the Sandwell consortium expressed considerable satisfaction with these. The carer profile asked carers to indicate the ways in which these services had been found to be helpful (Table 7). Most frequently mentioned were: having time now to do things for themselves, having someone to talk to, reliable care given to their dependants, and that receipt of the service made coping a bit easier (all these were described as 'very helpful' by nearly half the recipients of services). Also appreciated, by over a third, was the fact they now felt less stressed and anxious, and that their dependant now had a new interest and someone to talk to.

One of the central problems in the evaluation of carer services is the variety of services they provide. Since each scheme is giving a different kind of service, it is difficult, and potentially misleading, to make direct comparisons between them. Inevitably, carers using a service such as Sandwell Multi Handicap Group, who are receiving a regular sitting service, Saturday club and opportunity to attend a carer group, will feel 'helped' in more ways, than carers who used an information service, such as C.A.R.E.S., which might have been used only once, to obtain a particular piece of information. Yet both provide for different kinds of needs, and are, in important ways, complementary.

What is particularly striking (see Table 6) is the fact that carers found all services to be helpful in a variety of ways. C.A.R.E.S. and ICAN, with primary focus on advice, support and information to carers, were found to be particularly helpful in provision of information about services and benefits; however, a number of carers found other services helpful with information as well. All services were appreciated by at least a third of their carers because they gave them an opportunity to talk to someone about their situation, although Sandwell Multi-Handicap Group, with its carer group and Saturday club, scored particularly highly on this dimension. Akrill, as a day centre, was seen as particularly helpful by carers because it gave their relative an interest, yet even some of the carers using C.A.R.E.S. and ICAN, which were services directed at carer, rather than dependant needs, commented that they felt their dependants were helped by the service.

Inevitably, the services that provided regular respite care were the ones that were particularly appreciated for allowing the carer to have time to themselves, and very helpful in reducing stress and in helping carers to cope with their situation. However, a service like C.A.R.E.S. was also seen as having helped reduce stress and made coping easier, sometimes just because people knew that it was there if they needed information or someone to talk to, but also because the staff were not patronising and gave the information without making the carer feel guilty.

Carers were invited to comment on anything they particularly liked about the service they received. Most frequent comments were made about the friendliness and kindness of workers (16%) and how understanding and helpful these were (18%). Also appreciated was the fact that services were there when needed, even if the carer had not yet used them, that they were reliable and well organised (this comment was made particularly about Crossroads and the Multi-Handicap group care attendant services), and gave the carer peace of mind. Practical help to the carer, help in filling in forms and translating letters, was particularly appreciated by carers using the ICAN service.

Carers were invited also to comment on anything they didn't like about the services, or that made it difficult for them to use the schemes. Only 17 (5%) of carers made any criticism of the services they received, although a few (8) wrote that they had not used a service much, or had used it only for a short time so couldn't really comment. Some used this space to comment on their difficulties as carers, although not specifically criticising the service they received. The most frequent criticism of services were from carers (5) who would have liked more time, or who felt that there weren't enough workers to provide a more frequent service; a further three commented that a lack of back-up staff and resources meant that the services was not always available when they need it. One carer commented that the service didn't have anyone strong enough to cope with her dependant. A change in staff had caused difficulties for two carers: their dependants had got used to one helper and found it hard to adjust to another. Two carers criticised the meals that had been provided for their dependant and one carer had found the cost of day time phone calls a disincentive to using the telephone information service.

However, criticisms were few compared to the 222 favourable comments (70% of carers). Some of these comments suggest that the service, even if providing only a few hours each week, had made a profound difference to an extremely difficult situation, a few indicating that the situation may well have broken down without that help. The following quotes are not unrepresentative:

''It is a great help to know she is being cared for by kind people; it makes her so happy, and also me''

''The help I get from (sitting service) enables me to carry on working knowing that my wife is in capable hands''

''I've always seemed to cope until now, so I have been too proud to ask for help until I contacted (an advice and information service). Then I got help... you meet others who know how you feel when everything gets beyond you, and you can talk about it and not feel guilty.'' ''Nice to be able to live again''

''Nice to be able to accept wedding invitations again – I've been turning them down for years''

''Since we have been using this service it is though my husband and I have found each other again. We've had weekends alone, evenings out with no worries about our daughter''

''He would not be able to come home three days a week without this service''

For further information about the services described in this report contact Roger Page, Sandwell Carer Centre, 2 Bearwood Road, Smethwick. Telephone 021 558 7434.

Table 1 *Summary information on the eight services grant aided*

Scheme	Grant paid 1988/89	Other non-cash subsidies	Staffing	Services to carers
Sandwell Age Concern Home From Home – family placement for elderly people	£24183	Age Concern payroll and premises	2 part time organisers + host families	16 carers receive up to 2 weeks' respite
Akrill Day Centre (Sandwell) for elderly handicapped people	£14528 (cost of additional days opening)	SSD/church premises, SSD transport	1 part time staff + volunteers	4 day a week centre offers 7 hours p.w. to 45 fams.
The Sandcastle Project short-term fostering for handicapped children and young people	£19500 (part funded by SSD and Barnardos)	Barnardo's premises, supervision services payroll	Full time organiser + secretary + 2 field workers + host families	28 families receive respite: 2 hours to 2 weeks
C.A.R.E.S. Resource Centre for Carers providing phone line, information, advice and support, also carer group	£24286	Church premises	2 full time staff + volunteers	Service used by around 50 carers each month
Crossroads Care Attendant Scheme practical help and respite for wide range of carers	£50427	HA accom. National Crossroads training and support	2 Part time coordinators + care attendants	10–15 hours help per month per carer
Hately Heath Neighbourhood Visiting Scheme: voluntary support of elderly and handicapped	£2000	Support from Social Services	Volunteer co-ordinator, volunteer visitors	100 elderly and handicapped visited
I.C.A.N. (Sandwell) Asian Liaison scheme information and family support for Asian families with handicapped children	£12966	I.C.A.N. payroll, supervision, and accom. SSD second 2 staff as liaison workers	Full time social worker + 2 part time liaison workers	75 families supported

Table 1 *Summary information on the eight services grant aided* (Cont'd)

Scheme	Grant paid 1988/89	Other non-cash subsidies	Staffing	Services to carers
Sandwell Multi-handicap group sitting service Saturday club and carer group	£24890	Church premises	Full time coordinator and 16 part time care attendants	55 families receive around 20 hours relief per month

Table 2 *Carer profile Questionnaires: Response rate*

Scheme	Issued	Returned	%
Age Concern – Home from Home	15	13	87
Akrill Day Centre	50	20	40
Sandcastle	25	12	48
Hately Heath Neighbour Group	20	18	90
Sandwell M/H Group	85	55	65
Crossroads Care Att. Scheme	202	75	37
C.A.R.E.S.	339	75	22
I CAN	80	41	51
Total	736	332	45

* C.A.R.E.S. sent out a further 181 questionnaires to professional people and bodies, of which 30 were returned. However, these questionnaires were not included in the Carers Profile analysis.

Table 3 *Demographic characteristics of carers using grant aided services in Sandwell compared to carers in the General Household Survey.*

		Sandwell		GHS
Age of carer	16–29	7	02%	08%*
	30–44	103	34%	23%
	45–64	108	36%	43%
	64 and over	76	25%	26%
	(over 75)	(39	13%)	
	Not known	06	02%	
Sex of carer	men	63	21%	36%*
	women	199	66%	64%
	Not known	38	13%	

Table 3 *Demographic characteristics of carers using grant aided services in Sandwell compared to carers in the General Household Survey* (Cont'd)

		Sandwell		GHS
Marital status	married	211	73%	74%
	single	26	09%	14%
	widowed, divorced or separated	47	15%	12%
	not known	16	06%	
Relationship of dependant to carer	Spouse	98	33%	34%*
	Child	101	34%	18%
	parent (or parent in law)	74	25%	35%
	Other relative or friend	23	07%	12%
	not known	4	01%	
Where they live	Same house	247	83%	75%*
	next door	13	04%	
	further away	33	10%	
	hostel/institution	3	01%	25%
	other	1	01	
	not known	3	01%	
Age of dependant	0–4	17	06%	
	5–15	53	18%	10%**
	16–44	49	16%	16%
	45–64	30	10%	22%
	65–74	39	13%	18%
	75+	106	35%	33%
	not known	6	02%	
Sex of dependant	man	124	41%	36%**
	woman	158	53%	64%
	not known	18	06%	
Employment of Carer	full time	26	09%	26%*
	part time	25	09%	17%
	no paid	234	77%	57%
	not known	15	05%	
Length of time caring	Under 5 years	97	32%	46%**
	5–9 years	85	28%	25%
	10–14 years	57	19%	10%
	over 15 years	60	20%	8%
	not known	1	01%	

Table 3 *Demographic characteristics of carers using grant aided services in Sandwell compared to carers in the General Household Survey* (Cont'd)

		Sandwell		**GHS**
Number of hours a week spent caring	50 or more hours	207	69%	45%**
	20–49 hours	52	17%	17%
	under 20 hours	22	07%	37%
	not known	19	07%	
Dependant is suffering from	Physical disability	144	48%	67%**
	Mental disability	37	12%	9%
	Physical and mental disability	64	21%	22%
	Old age			1%
	No information	34	12%	
What kind of care:				
a) help with personal care		261	87%	53%**
b) help with paper work/ finances		233	78%	47%
c) practical help		296	99%	82%
d) keeping company		289	96%	64%
e) taking out		240	82%	47%
f) giving medicine		255	85%	46%
g) keeping an eye		293	98%	69%
Can dependant be left alone?				
Could leave without someone sitting		90	30%	65%**
Couldn't leave without sitter		201	67%	35%
Not known		9	03%	35%
Carer would find arranging a sitter				
	very difficult	96	31%	8%**
	quite difficult	83	28%	7%
	not very difficult	59	20%	20%
	haven't tried	49	16%	65%
	not known	13	04%	

*,**, Sandwell figures are compared with figures taken from tables in the General Household Survey referring to (*) carers who were caring for over 20 hours per week or (**) carers who were caring for someone in their own household. Most of the Sandwell carers came into both these categories.

Table 3A *Characteristics of carers using different schemes*

	SCHEME						
	Age Conc.	**Akril**	**Crossrds**	**SMH**	**ICAN**	**Barn**	**CARES**
Relationship spouse	37%	48%	50%				30%
child			1%	88%	100%	100%	35%
parent	50%	45%	39%				31%
relative		4%	6%	9%			7%
friend		2%					1%
Lives in same house	75%	88%	75%	86%	97%	100%	82%
next door	12%	12%	4%	4%			2%
other			20%	9%			14%
Mean yrs caring	12	9	6	14	8	11	9
Helping under 20hrs	12%	8%	6%	2%	10%	—	7%
20–49hrs	12%	12%	17%	11%	18%	—	26%
Over 50hrs	75%	72%	67%	77%	65%	100%	66%
Helps with personal care	88%	76%	88%	94%	97%	100%	85%
Could leave	37%	56%	35%	6%	5%	—	46%
Can't leave	62%	40%	64%	88%	89%	100%	58%
Finding sitter would be							
very difficult	25%	32%	39%	32%	42%	16%	25%
quite difficult	37%	8%	30%	37%	18%	50%	25%
not very difficult	25%	24%	16%	23%	18%	25%	20%
haven't tried	12%	32%	12%	—	5%	—	28%
Sex male		36%	33%	11%	8%	—	25%
female	88%	48%	59%	73%	76%	100%	66%
Age carer							
16–19	—	—			16%		
20–44		20%	22%	51%	38%	83%	21%
45–64	62%	48%	31%	36%	13%	16%	51%
65–74	25%	12%	21%	6%			14%
75+	12%	20%	25%	4%			1%
Age dependant							
0–14	—	—		15%	18%	8%	1%
5–15	—	—	1%	30%	65%	66%	4%
16–44	—	—	7%	45%	16%	25%	14%
45–64	12%	16%	1%	10%	—	—	25%
65–74	—	16%	26%	—	—	—	19%
75+	88%	68%	65%	—	—	—	37%
Dependant male	37%	40%	35%	43%	37%	66%	46%
female	50%	60%	63%	47%	47%	25%	50%
Carer works							
full time		8%	16%	4%			11%
part time		8%	8%	6%	5%	8%	12%
no paid work	100%	80%	74%	79%	89%	92%	75%

Table 4 *Problems experienced by carers using funded services*

Problems	Number who found it a constant problem						
	Age Concern	Akrill	Cross-roads	CARES	Barn-ardos	ICAN	SMH
Laundry	2 25%	3 12%	21 28%	15 18%	6 50%	11 29%	16 30%
Housecleaning	4 50%	7 28%	22 29%	30 36%	5 42%	11 29%	16 30%
Lifting	4 50%	5 20%	27 35%	21 25%	4 33%	12 32%	26 49%
Bathing	3 37%	8 32%	29 38%	24 28%	5 42%	14 37%	25 47%
Health	3 37%	6 24%	34 44%	39 46%	5 42%	8 21%	17 32%
Own time	3 37%	11 44%	37 48%	30 36%	7 58%	16 42%	24 45%
Getting out	3 37%	6 24%	37 48%	29 34%	3 25%	16 42%	18 34%
Keeping in touch	2 25%	3 12%	20 26%	25 29%	5 42%	11 29%	15 28%
Strain in family	0 —	4 16%	15 19%	22 26%	4 16%	11 29%	15 28%
Worry future	4 50%	12 48%	34 45%	44 52%	7 58%	30 79%	37 69%
Lack of sleep	2 25%	8 32%	32 42%	36 43%	5 42%	15 39%	18 34%
Stress	3 37%	6 24%	37 48%	48 57%	8 66%	16 42%	27 51%
Behaviour dep	4 50%	2 8%	19 25%	15 18%	3 25%	10 26%	17 32%
No one	0 —	2 8%	11 14%	20 24%	2 21%	7 18%	14 26%
Money	2 25%	7 28%	11 14%	15 18%	6 50%	10 26%	12 23%
Doubts	3 37%	6 24%	15 19%	20 24%	1 8%	12 32%	8 15%
Where help	1 12%	7 28%	13 17%	20 24%	2 21%	10 26%	10 19%
House	2 25%	1 4%	3 4%	13 15%	3 25%	13 34%	9 17%

Table 5 *Sources of help for Carers*

	Number indicating service received	as % carers responding to questionnaire
Aids and adaptations (bath aids, walker etc)	189	63%
Major adaptations	96	32%
Home help	111	37%
Meals on wheels	35	12%
Nurse (community nurse, health visitor)	132	44%

Table 5 *Sources of help for Carers* (Cont'd)

	Number indicating service received	**as % carers responding to questionnaire**
Occupational therapist	48	16%
Laundry service	42	14%
Physiotherapist	59	20%
Sitting or relief care service	137	45%
Respite care (in home or hospital)	94	31%
Day centre or day hospital	119	40%
School or adult training centre	89	30%
Social worker/welfare officer	127	42%
GP	219	73%
Hospital Consultant	146	48%
Community Psychiatric Nurse	36	12%
Carer support group	136	45%
Counsellor or psychologist	39	13%
Benefits like ICA, attendance allowance etc	224	75%
A voluntary organisation	77	26%
Friends or neighbours	174	58%
Family	184	61%

Table 5A *Carers who received help found it:*

	very helpful	**quite helpful**	**not very helpful**	**Total in receipt**
Aids and adaptations (bath aids, walker etc)	51%	36%	13%	189
Major adaptations	59%	22%	19%	96
Home help	62%	28%	9%	111
Meals on wheels	40%	14%	46%	35
Nurse (community nurse, health visitor)	54%	31%	15%	132
Occupational therapist	37%	26%	37%	48
Laundry service	50%	21%	29%	42

Table 5A *Carers who received help found it:* (Cont'd)

	very helpful	quite helpful	not very helpful	Total in receipt
Physiotherapist	51%	22%	27%	59
Sitting or relief care service	75%	22%	3%	137
Respite care (in a home or hospital)	67%	9%	14%	94
Day centre or day hospital	63%	27%	10%	119
School or adult training centre	75%	18%	7%	89
Social worker/welfare officer	49%	33%	18%	127
GP	54%	36%	10%	219
Hospital Consultant	44%	40%	16%	146
Community Psychiatric Nurse	28%	31%	41%	36
Carer support group	73%	11%	6%	136
Counsellor or psychologist	36%	18%	46%	39
Benefits like ICA, attendance allowance etc	80%	19%	1%	224
A voluntary organisation	84%	16%	0%	77
Friends or neighbours	40%	35%	25%	174
Family	49%	16%	25%	184

Table 6 *Ways in which carers felt helped by funded schemes*

Percentage of all carers reporting schemes to be helpful in the following ways:

Type of help	Percentage finding service		
	Very helpful	Quite helpful	Not helpful/ doesn't apply*
1. Physical help, like lifting and dressing	20	8	72
2. Time to yourself, time to do other things	45	13	42
3. Information about other services and benefits	29	17	54
4. Information about your relative/friend's illness, handicap and how to manage this	16	10	74
5. Someone to talk to	45	16	39
6. Helped you feel less stressed and anxious	37	21	42

Table 6 *Ways in which carers felt helped by funded schemes* Cont'd

Type of help	**Percentage finding service**		
	Very helpful	**Quite helpful**	**Not helpful/ doesn't apply***
7. Helped you meet others with similar problems	20	12	68
8. Gave reliable care to relative/friend	33	11	56
9. Gave relative/friend an interest, someone to talk to	36	11	53
10. Made coping a bit easier	47	17	36
Total number		308	

* The questionnaire asked all carers if they found their service helpful on all these dimensions, even if it was not immediately relevant, as in the case of an information service for carers, giving their dependant an interest and someone to talk to. What was surprising was the number of carers that said that their service was helpful on a number of dimensions which did not, at first seem to be relevant, suggesting that the voluntary services provided a range of assistance, outside of their original brief.

Table 7 *Ways in which carers felt helped by the 7 funded schemes*

	Age Concern		**Akrill**		**Sand-castle**		**SMHG**		**Cross-roads**		**CARES**		**I CAN**	
	VH %	QH %	VH %	QH %	VH %	QH %	VH %	QH %	VH %	QH %	VH %	QH %	VH %	QH %
Helped with physical tasks	15	—	21	17	25	8	49	13	14	6	4	4	10	4
Information benefits	23	7	21	16	16	17	20	25	10	10	43	12	59	19
Someone to talk to	38	7	33	16	42	16	71	18	25	11	32	6	61	15
Met others	—	15	32	16	42	16	43	18	2	3	15	—	22	15
Gave relative interest	38	—	67	17	33	16	36	13	32	8	19	9	19	21
Time to self	46	—	46	33	67	16	76	9	40	8	7	7	41	20
Information illness	15	—	8	12	16	8	18	14	5	5	16	5	29	15
Less stressed	27	—	29	37	16	16	60	22	27	12	17	13	46	24

Printed in the United Kingdom for
HMSO Dd 290371 C50 2/91